KU-747-072

Sheila Kitzinger helps you write your own book about your experiences of pregnancy and after

SHEILA KITZINGER is a childbirth educator and social anthropologist who studies birth in different cultures. She works with the National Childbirth Trust in Britain and is on its Panel of Advisors. She is also a Consultant for the International Childbirth Education Association. She lectures widely in North and South America, Europe, South Africa and Australia. ●Her previous books include: *The Experience of Childbirth* (Penguin), *The Place of Birth* (OUP), *The Good Birth Guide* (Fontana), *Giving Birth: Emotions in Childbirth* (Sphere), *Birth at Home* (OUP), *The Experience of Breastfeeding* (Penguin), *Women as Mothers* (Fontana), *Education and Counselling for Childbirth* (Baillière Tindall). ●She and her husband Uwe have five daughters and live in the country near Oxford.

SUZANNE ARMS is a photographer and author whose special interest lies in family life and relationships at the time of birth. She is also a consumer advocate, a lecturer in childbirth, and has spoken widely in North America, Canada, England and Australia. She is a founder of The Birth Place, a community-owned-and-operated birth home and resource centre. ●She lives with her family in Portola Valley, California.

Sheila Kitzinger's BIRTH BOOK

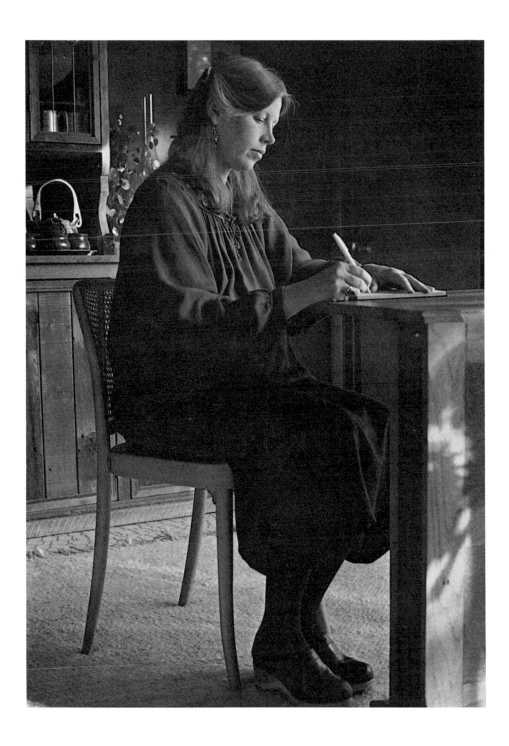

Sheila Kitzinger's
BIRTH
BOOK

A JOURNAL OF YOUR THOUGHTS

AND FEELINGS ABOUT CHILDBIRTH

With photographs by

Suzanne Arms

FONTANA PAPERBACKS

First published by Fontana Paperbacks
in association with Heinrich Hanau, 1980.

Text copyright © 1980 Sheila Kitzinger.

All photographs copyright © Suzanne Arms 1980,
with exception of photograph on page 29 which is
reproduced by permission of John David Arms. Photographs
appearing on pages 113, 114 and 119–20 are from the film
Five Women-Five Births copyright © Suzanne Arms 1978.

Design and typography by Anthony Frewin.
Composed on the Monotype in Grotesque, Series 215,
by Avontype, Bristol, England, and printed
and bound in the United States of America.

Conditions of Sale
This book is sold subject to the condition that
it shall not, by way of trade or otherwise, be lent,
re-sold, hired out or otherwise circulated without the
publisher's prior consent in any form of binding or cover
other than that in which it is published and without
a similar condition including this condition
being imposed on the subsequent purchaser.

Contents

Each week is accompanied by a page
on which to record your own
reflections and observations.
You might wish to put in some
photographs of your own.

The first signs that you are expecting
a child usually come after you are
about six weeks pregnant (i.e. you
have missed your first period and
probably conceived about two weeks
after your last period). So the book
starts at six weeks and then, since
things are still very uncertain in the
first weeks, skips to eight weeks, ten,
and twelve weeks, and from then on,
with the pregnancy firmly established,
the book goes week by week.

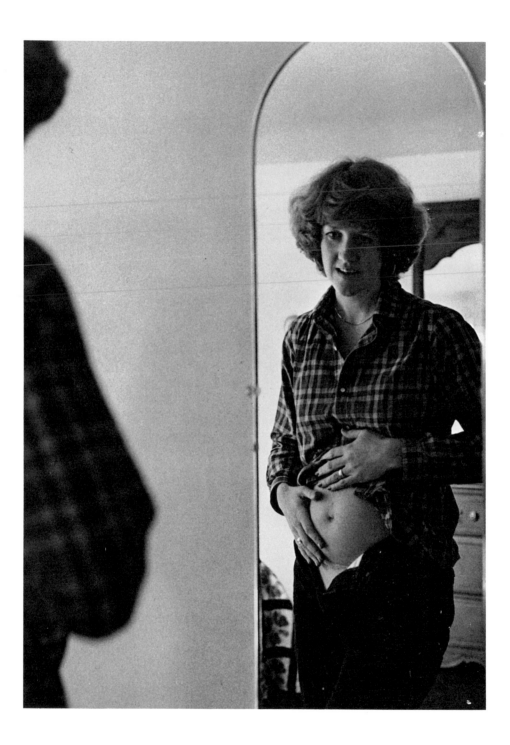

A Note to the Reader

Pregnancy is not only a waiting time. It is a time for physical and emotional preparation for the birth and for being parents. This book is designed to help you during the journey. There is plenty of instruction available for pregnant women, telling us what we ought to do and what happens to us, but very little about what it *feels* like to have a baby growing inside, and relatively little too about what it *feels* like to get to know your new baby and be confronted and astonished by its developing personality. •Acquiring information and doing exercises is one way of preparing. But it is not enough. Education for birth is not really like training for an athletic event or learning skills like those for driving a car. It is more a matter of learning to know and understand your body, enjoying its changing shape and its new curves. Another vital aspect is learning more about yourself and your emotions. Neither of these things can be done all at once. They take time. Fortunately pregnancy lasts nine months. There is ample opportunity for this unfolding, this process of self-discovery and awareness. •Here then is a book to be a companion through your pregnancy and the three months after birth which can stimulate you to reflect, think and feel, a book which is also a record in which you can make notes about what the experience means to you. •In some ways you are more fully alive in pregnancy because there is another life deep inside you. And after the birth too, especially through breastfeeding, your body is irrevocably linked with the life of the new baby. •The point of this book is to help you feel enriched by that intensified life of your body – and the often startling and difficult, but always exciting, first steps over the bridge into motherhood. •In the years to come when your child wants to talk with you about his or her birth, this record of your ideas and emotions during pregnancy and in the weeks after birth can provide a focus for your discussion about the child's journey to life and your own psychological journey to motherhood. •A pregnant woman creates the environment for her developing baby as it grows, weightless and floating, like an astronaut in space, in the fluid inside the amniotic sac. The baby is automatically shielded from bumps, kept at an even temperature and protected from harmful bacteria, and can easily exercise its limbs in the mother's inner sea. •The placenta, a tree of life for the baby, filters nutrients and oxygen from your bloodstream into the umbilical cord and straight into the baby's bloodstream. Waste products flow from the baby in the other direction, pass through the placenta into your circulatory system and are excreted. • The placenta strains out many things which could harm the baby, but some harmful substances can pass through the placenta, including numerous drugs, nicotine, and alcohol. •This is why the way you care for yourself and your life-style during pregnancy are so important. The food you eat, the air you breathe, medicines you take, the powerful emotions you experience, all can affect the baby in subtle ways. You want to give the baby the best start in life, a protected environment in the uterus. The way to do this is to look after yourself and provide the best nutrition and the happiest emotional setting for pregnancy. •When you drug yourself you drug your baby. Throw away all medicines which have not been prescribed for pregnancy. Discuss with your doctor those about which you are doubtful. If you take any over-the-counter drug, even just something for indigestion or heartburn, ask the chemist or your doctor whether it is recommended for use in pregnancy and read the small print in the package insert before taking it. •If you have nausea or morning sickness, nibble a few biscuits or some dry toast and sip a cup of tea or a glass of hot water before you get out of bed in the morning. Eat something every two to three hours and avoid fatty foods. When you have a headache or any other pain lie down in a darkened room and see if you can sleep it off rather than taking medicine. If you are uncomfortable, tired, or lie awake at night, adjust your daily life, cut back on some activities, eat small, frequent meals instead of larger ones, drink extra fluids, add fibres to your diet, use extra pillows so that you can sleep propped up, lie down for half an hour before or after a meal and practice controlled relaxation and rhythmic breathing. •If no pregnant woman ever smoked this alone would do more than anything else to save babies' lives. Smoking is the single major element in our polluted environment which we ourselves could eradicate for the sake of our babies. •Smoking more than five cigarettes a day increases the risk of losing your baby through miscarriage or stillbirth. Some babies of smoking mothers are born prematurely because they are literally starved in the uterus. Many others are of low birth weight and need special care. Not only does nicotine constrict the blood vessels in the cord and placenta, but carbon monoxide in the mother's bloodstream reduces the oxygen available in the blood that does reach the baby. •The more a woman smokes, the more the baby is likely to be affected. •There is some evidence that the *father*'s smoking also affects the baby, even if the mother does not smoke, and that breathing in other people's tobacco smoke can be harmful. In one research study fathers who smoked had more children who were premature and the prematurity rate increased with the amount the fathers smoked.

Sheila Kitzinger

Sheila Kitzinger's BIRTH BOOK

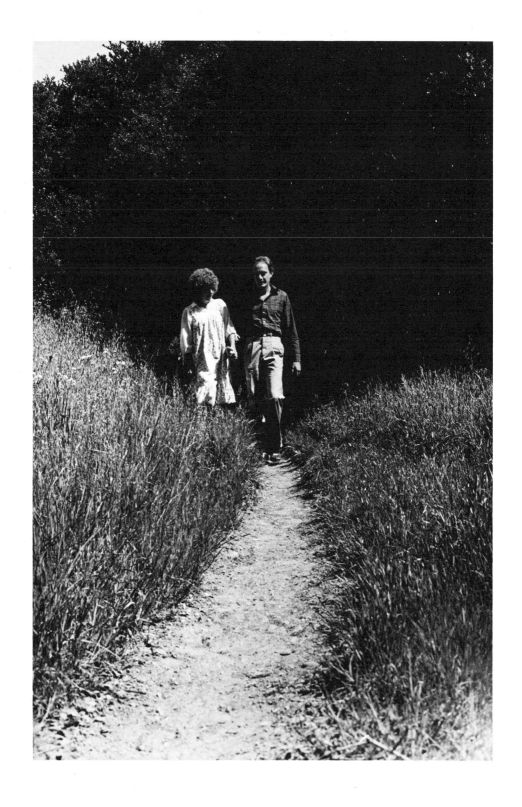

Around Six Weeks

Pregnant? •Odd things are happening to your body which are difficult to understand and make you feel that it has 'taken over'. •The first sign of being pregnant is probably a missed period, but about one third of pregnant women have bleeding which looks like a very small period instead. There may be other signs of pregnancy though. Nausea is common, especially in the early morning or late afternoon; some women have it all day. You may not be able to tolerate fatty, fried food and find that you get a digestive upset after a heavy meal. •Nine out of ten women experience inexplicable tiredness in the first three months and long to sleep undisturbed for hours on end. If you can sleep the clock round and wake up only to go back to sleep again in a few hours you may discover that this is the best treatment not only for the exhaustion you feel but for nausea too, since it is made much worse by tiredness. You won't go on feeling like this right through your pregnancy. Your body is making the first, and major, adjustment to pregnancy. •You may feel a strange, aching tenderness in your breasts, and they often throb. They are changing, ready for feeding your baby later. They swell and the network of veins gets more pronounced, like rivers on a map. The circle round your nipple has become darker and the little brown bumps more prominent. •You may not yet be absolutely sure you are pregnant. Many doctors do not 'confirm' a pregnancy till you have missed two periods. But a pregnancy test is likely to give you an accurate result now. Even then, you can't help wondering whether your next period will suddenly turn up and it will have been all a dream. •Thinking about being pregnant may produce mixed emotions too, delight, elation perhaps, but also something approaching panic. If you have been trying for a baby for a long time you will feel a sense of triumph, but many women become pregnant before they have made a definite decision about wanting a baby and if you come off the Pill 'to see what happens', as many do, the thought that you have actually got pregnant may astonish and even alarm you. It can be a shock to discover that you are capable of conceiving. Many women secretly feel that they can't. The emotional impact of all this may mean that you can't help feeling tense and anxious, even though you want the baby. •It will probably be in the middle of the night when you think 'Will everything be all right? . . . What if I can't stand the pain? . . . Will the baby be normal? . . . Can I cope when the baby comes?' Ann Oakley revealed in *Women*

Confined (London, 1980), that nearly 40% of pregnant women worried that they might have a deformed baby, 35% were anxious about giving up work and the change in life-style, 32% had fears about labour, 29% about losing the baby and 20% about money or housing. The chances are that you have several of these worries. All the evidence goes to show that it is normal to experience all these conflicting feelings. •This is the time when your unborn baby, still a tiny speck of potential life deep inside your uterus, is most affected by toxic substances. Avoid all drugs. •At this stage toxic substances pass readily to the tiny embryo and can have major effects. •The embryo's head is very large in relation to the rest of its body at this stage of development. It is still less than the top joint of your finger. It looks like a miniature seahorse, with the upper end curled round and top heavy, though already the face is beginning to have human features, with big, open eyes, a flat nose rather like a little snout, an overhanging brow and not much chin.

Around Six Weeks

Reflections & Observations

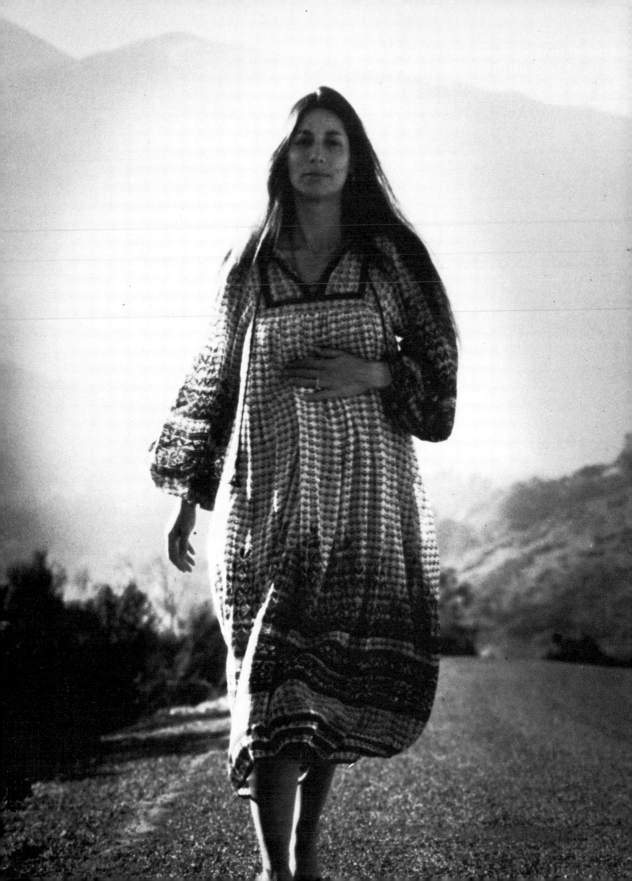

About Eight Weeks

Yes, pregnant! •It is exciting to be pregnant, yet you may feel disappointed that you don't feel more vibrant, but still be patient if you can. Things will get easier later. Your whole metabolism is adjusting to the life growing inside you. About this time, too, you may feel some low backache and heaviness in your pelvis as if you are about to have a period. Many women experience this, but the period never comes. However, it is a sign that you could do with some extra rest when your period would have been due. •It may still be difficult to believe that you really are pregnant, but there is one sign that becomes increasingly more persuasive: pressure from the enlarging uterus may mean that you need to empty your bladder often. •This is a time when you especially value close holding, physical tenderness and acceptance from a partner who is calm, loving and constant. Any anxiety he expresses, questions such as 'Have you taken your iron today? Are you sure?' or insistence that you must put your feet up, prove extremely irritating. You may snap at him. On the other hand, if he seems to ignore the fact that you are pregnant, that can be hurtful too. So he may have to steer a careful course between being over-solicitous and apparently neglectful. •The embryo is looking more human and is about the size of a prune. The trunk has plumped out so that though the head is still the largest part there is now a firm little pot-belly under it. Arms and legs are short and stumpy and tucked up in front of the body like a kitten's paws; fingers and toes are just budding. All the main organs of the body have now been formed. •What were your feelings when you first realized you actually were pregnant?

About Eight Weeks

Reflections & Observations

About Ten Weeks

It is disconcerting, just as you are adjusting to the idea of your pregnancy and are probably beginning to accept being pregnant as normal and natural, to be turned into a *patient*. •Since in the West today pregnancy is first and foremost a medical condition you will probably discover that doctors emphasize the dangers of childbirth. Pregnancy can be turned into a kind of obstacle race against high blood pressure, putting on too much weight, not gaining enough weight, dates queried and so on. •Though a pregnant woman in our society is usually expected to hand over responsibility for her own body, you can make it clear to your doctor from the first that you want to take responsibility for yourself and your baby. You can do this by asking questions, listening to the answers and asking further questions if you do not feel sufficiently well informed, and by finding out all you can about pregnancy and birth and how you can work *with* your body rather than fighting it. •Even while you are still getting used to the fact that you are really going to have a baby there are important decisions that have to be made about where and how you want to give birth. Many women leave these decisions with the doctor. Others want to decide for themselves. If this is how you feel, tell your doctor that you would like to discuss alternatives as to the place of birth and the way labour is conducted. When you have had a talk take a little time to think it over, since it can be difficult to change your obstetrician or to change from hospital to home, for example, later in pregnancy. •If doctors and nurses talk in front of you or over your body about things you don't understand or find worrying, ask them to explain. If you don't do this you will carry the anxiety with you till your next visit and in the interval it tends to be magnified, and each word and phrase which gave rise to mild apprehension grows into a threat which can destroy your peace of mind.

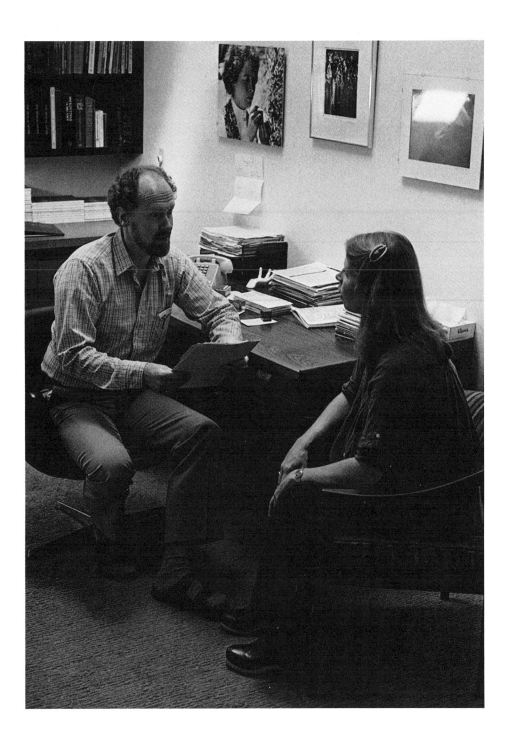

About Ten Weeks

Reflections & Observations

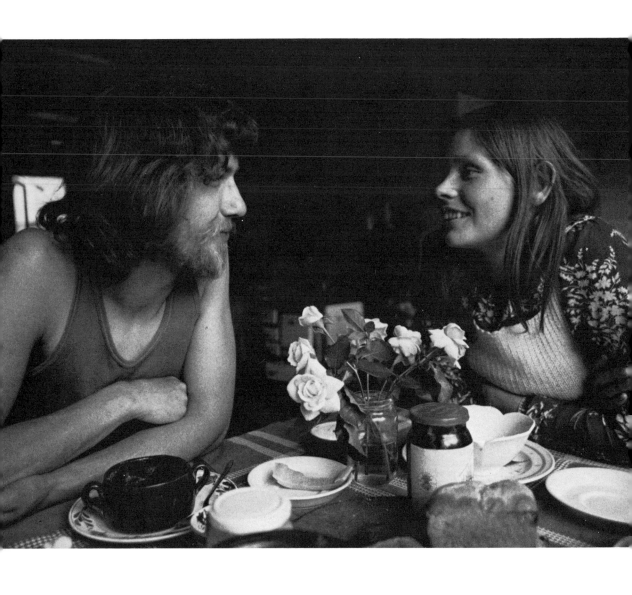

Twelve Weeks

Having a baby is not just something that happens to you; it can be something you actively do yourself. It is worth finding out what options are available and making decisions about how you would like the birth to be. Bear in mind that all plans must be provisional. Here are some of the things you may want to discuss together:

- Do you want to be together for the birth?
- Home or hospital?
- If hospital, would you prefer a highpowered one with all the sophisticated modern technology or a smaller, simpler one? If home, who will attend the birth?
- Do you hope to have a natural (prepared) birth or not? If so, to which classes will you go?
- Do you plan on having drugs for pain relief? Pethidine and sometimes tranquillizers are given by injection; gas and oxygen you administer yourself through a mask; an epidural, given in your lower spine, may be used to freeze the lower part of your body. The anaesthetic works much like an injection used at the dentist's. Would you like complete eradication of sensation for as long as possible or do you want to retain some feeling? Do you value emotional support for pain relief? Remember that all drugs introduced into your bloodstream go through to your baby.
- Do you want to have control over any drugs and medical procedures done to you?
- After the birth do you want to have your baby with you all the time while you are in hospital, or would you prefer it to be in the nursery for some of the time?
- Discuss all these things with your doctor or midwife too and ask him or her about any possible effects on you and your baby of different choices.

•You are now over that part of pregnancy when miscarriages are common. Though past the stage when toxic drugs do most harm, the way you live, the substances you take into your body, how you respond to stress and deal with challenges can all affect your baby, even though indirectly. It is a good idea to look at your life-style to see how you can provide the best environment for the developing fetus. •Your uterus is now about the size of a satsuma and is still pressing close to your bladder. The baby, at first called an embryo, is a *fetus* from now on. It is about the size of your index finger and is complete in miniature. It can kick, move its mouth, swallow and turn its head. Even at this early stage the sex of the baby can be distinguished and from now on babies begin to look different from each other. •Though the pregnancy is now a certainty, there are many unknown things in the future. You will be thinking forward to the time after the baby comes and trying to make up your mind whether or not to return to work outside the home and, if so, whether it should be sooner or later. Having a first baby is such a major transformation in a woman's life that it raises fundamental questions about your personal goals and satisfactions, the way you see your role as a woman and your ideas about the baby's emotional needs. There are no easy solutions to all this. Though you may feel that you slot into being a mother with no difficulty and that this is what you want most of all, it isn't like that for many women. Share these thoughts with other women who already have children since they can help you sort out your priorities.

Twelve Weeks

Reflections & Observations

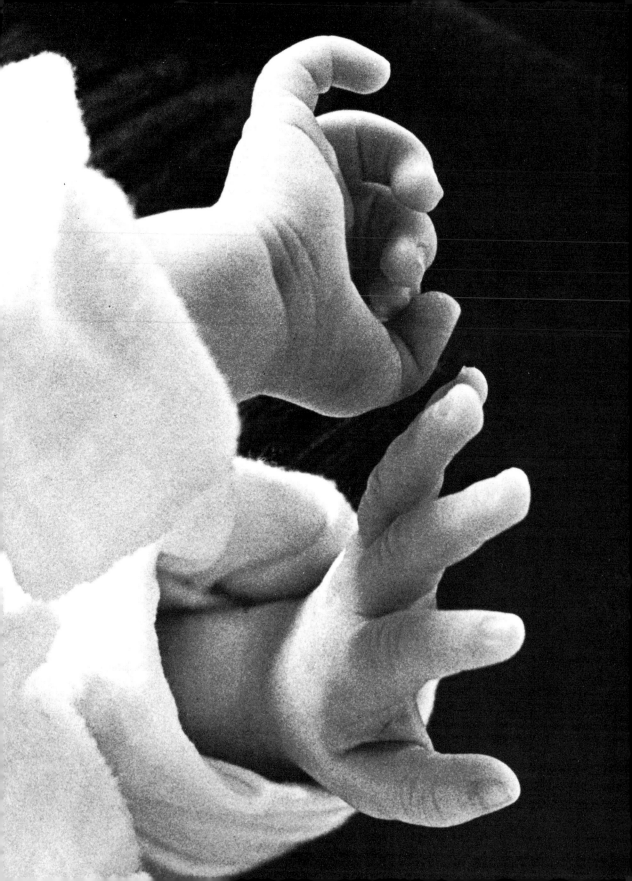

Thirteen Weeks

Although you are not yet aware of your baby's movements, it is exercising its limbs, bouncing around your uterus like an astronaut in space, attached by its umbilical cord to the placenta, its life support system. The spine and rib cage have hardened and the arms are in correct proportion to the rest of the tiny body. Even the budding nails are just visible. Each toe is clearly differentiated. The baby can now make delicate movements of hands and feet, curling its toes, clenching fists, opening its hands and moving the wrists. •The eyes are tightly closed now and remain so until ten or twelve weeks before birth. The ova and sperms which will mature at puberty are already beginning to develop inside the baby's body. •The placenta is the tree of life for the baby. Its exterior surface is bathed in pools of your blood, but separated from them by a fine membrane, through which oxygen and nutrients filter through into the baby's bloodstream and across which waste products from the baby can filter back again into your blood. •As well as feeding the baby and removing its waste, the placenta protects it from illnesses to which you are yourself immune and from the effect of many drugs and other toxic substances. It also manufactures hormones which keep the pregnancy going, help your body to make major adjustments to serve the developing life inside you, and which at the end of pregnancy trigger off labour.

Thirteen Weeks

Reflections & Observations

Fourteen Weeks

What is a baby really like and how does it feel to be parents? You begin to see your friends who already have children in a new light. You notice how they handle their babies and think ahead to how you plan to be with your child. •This is a time when any tiredness and nausea you have felt has probably disappeared and you are fit and energetic again. This is a good time too for starting some simple exercises for your pelvic floor muscles. These are shaped like a figure '8' round your vagina and rectum and other layers of muscle are angled like slanting stage scenery further up inside. At the front, they are attached to your pubic bone. Feel it just above your clitoris. They stretch across to the bones at the bottom of your spine. These muscles support your bladder and uterus and so need to have good tone to take the added weight of pregnancy. In labour they open up so that the baby can slide down to be born. •If these muscles are weak you will find urine leaking when you cough, sneeze, or laugh. But it is not just a matter of avoiding a weak pelvic floor. Well-toned muscles enrich lovemaking: as you contract them they make a 'kiss inside' during intercourse. There are nerve endings in these muscles which are a source of sexual pleasure. So increasing your awareness of and ability to use them can make intercourse more satisfying. •Think of the muscles as a lift. You are going to gradually tighten them as if the lift is moving from the ground up to the fourth floor. (Go on breathing!) When you reach the third floor you will already feel a good deal of pressure against your bladder. Now tighten and pull the muscles up even more. (Don't try and do it with your shoulders.) Further still. Hold for four or five seconds and then go down, little by little, till you reach the ground floor again. Then go down to the basement, push downward and outward, bulging out the muscles. This is the essence of pushing and is what you will do in labour when you are ready to push your baby out. It is not a great athletic event, but simply a release and movement down and forward of all the muscles of your pelvic floor. Now finish by going up to the first floor again, so that you complete the exercise with a toning action. It is a good idea to do this whenever you go upstairs, when you wait at the checkout at the supermarket or for the lights to change, and at other times when you have to stand around. •Think of the ring of muscles about halfway up inside your vagina as like a mouth which is capable of many different expressions. You will find that you can actually 'smile' with your pelvic floor. Each morning when you wake up greet the day with a pelvic floor smile! And just as you talk with your mouth you will discover that you can 'talk' with your pelvic floor, mobilising it fully and so toning it. Having a pelvic floor which is 'alive' is not just a matter of exercises at set times but of being aware of this part of your body and making it as expressive as the muscles of your face. It may sound an odd task to undertake, but in fact these muscles are probably the most important muscles in a woman's body and your well-being and vitality depend on their good tone. •By now your baby is capable of different facial expressions and sometimes frowns. You still don't feel any kicking because there is a good deal of space in the uterus around the tiny body. The baby is now sucking and swallowing inside you, drinking the fluid in which it floats and passing it through its digestive system and kidneys. It is also making breathing movements, using muscles which will later draw in oxygen and exhale carbon dioxide, though now the breathing passages are bathed in amniotic fluid.

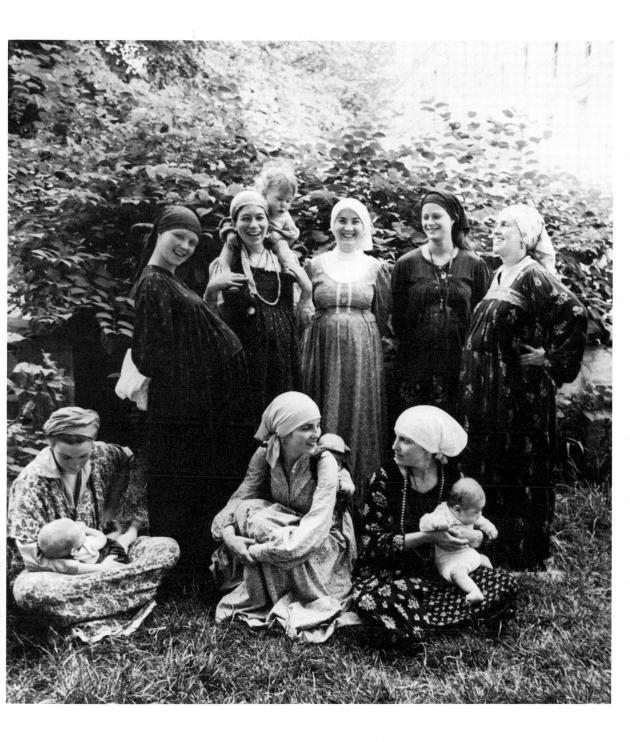

Fourteen Weeks

Reflections & Observations

Fifteen Weeks

'But do I have any maternal instincts? How do I know that I am capable of being a mother? I don't know anything about babies. Help!' •Many women feel like this, and it is a more realistic approach to motherhood than being sure that you are going to take it all in your stride. Even people like nurses and doctors who work with children find it is very different when they have their own babies. Each person has to start from the beginning to get to know her or his own child. •Watch other women with their babies. Talk with new parents to discover what the experience is like for them. If you can, 'borrow' a mother with her new baby for a day. She will show you how she feeds, changes nappies and copes with bathtime, and it will give you a chance to handle a tiny baby. •If you are alone, without the support of a partner, this kind of contact is particularly important. Reach out to get the help you need. •Discover the resources in your community. There may be a group for one-parent families or another self-help group through which you can be in touch with others who have been through a similar experience. •Even if you have a partner's support, if you have recently moved into a community you may be feeling very out of touch. Next time you go out do a bit of detective work and see if you can find out what is going on, groups you can join and people you can meet. Explore available help and fellowship by investigating through local women's organisations, the church and the community centre and look for notices in your public library.

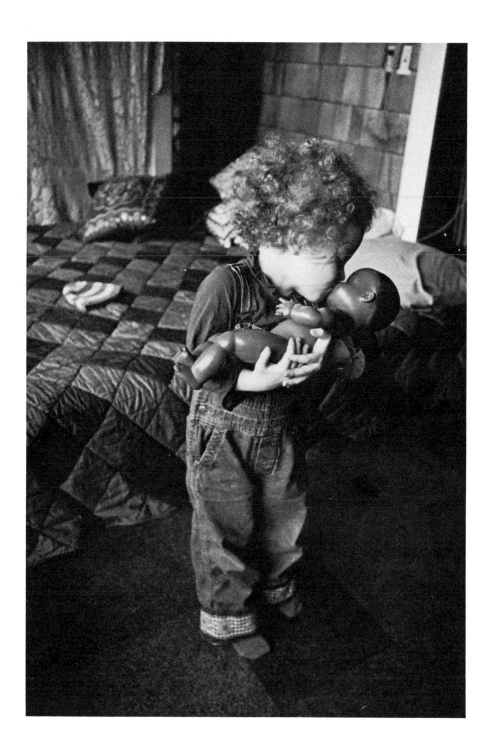

Fifteen Weeks

Reflections & Observations

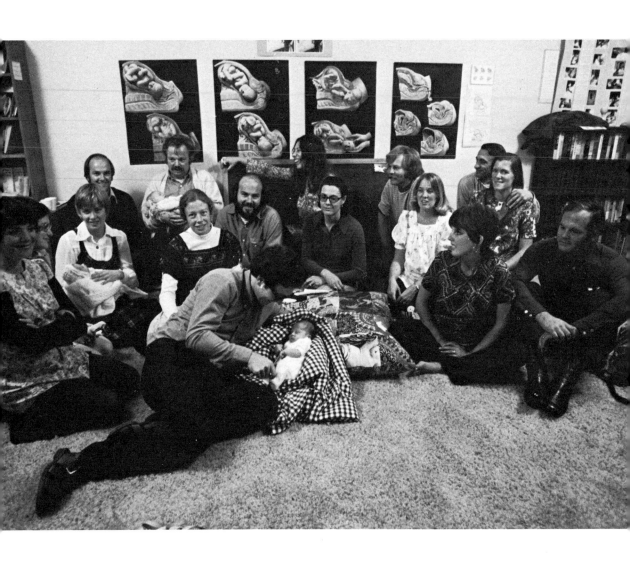

Sixteen Weeks

By now you have probably read some books about birth and registered for child-birth education classes. If not, it is a good time to do so. You will have more knowledge about what it is like to have a baby and will have your own ideas about the kind of care you prefer. You can read about some things which you may want to discuss with your doctor too including some practices which many parents are now questioning. ●One is induction and acceleration of labour with an oxytocin intravenous drip. In this way labour can be started off at the most convenient time or augmented so that it doesn't last long. There are clear medical reasons for inducing sometimes, such as diabetes or pre-eclamptic toxaemia, or when the baby is not being adequately nourished by the placenta. At other times induction is not essential. Disadvantages are that the baby may not be ready to be born just yet, that you can't walk around in labour, and that contractions may be fast and furious. How do you feel about this? ●Shaving of your pubic hair and an enema or suppositories are routine practices performed on admission in most hospitals. Neither is essential. ●Many hospitals artificially rupture the membranes on admission too if labour is established. You don't have to have it done if you would rather not. ●Fifty-per-cent of women or more now have episiotomy at delivery. This is a cut to enlarge the birth opening. It is usually done to speed up the birth and to take pressure off the mother's perineal tissues. If you don't want it done unless it is essential, say so. ●It is usually just a matter of time before the baby is born and if you only push as hard as you want to and *not a bit stronger or longer* the tissues of your perineum are likely to fan out gradually. ●Now your baby is about 12 cm. long, the same size as its placenta. From now on it is a matter of growth and development of organs which already exist rather than the creation of new ones. The vocal chords have developed so that if it were not immersed in amniotic fluid it could cry. Fine hairs called lanugo cover the body and a protective cream, vernix, like curd-cheese, clings to the skin and prevents it from getting too wrinkled by the water. Already your baby has its finger-print, different from everybody else's.

Sixteen Weeks

Reflections & Observations

Seventeen Weeks

Increased blood flows to your pelvic area and the weight of the enlarged uterus pressing on your pelvic muscles and vagina may make you enjoy sex very much in mid-pregnancy. At least this is how it is with some women – not at all with others. Sometimes pelvic pain or tingling results if you get sexually excited without experiencing climax, for the pelvis is temporarily engorged. Tender lovemaking is a normal part of the middle weeks of pregnancy though some couples are happier not having intercourse right through pregnancy. Your uterus may contract rhythmically after orgasm and you feel this because it is now so large. Provided it does not hurt and you do not get any bleeding after intercourse, there is no reason to think that the baby can be harmed by gentle, loving sex. The baby is protected in the amniotic sea and may experience the contractions as pulsing movements in the fluid in which it is bathed. •Exercise in the fresh air is important in pregnancy and benefits both you and the baby. Walking and swimming are some of the best forms because they encourage good circulation, involve rhythmic movement of the whole body and do not cause strain. Competitive sports are not suitable for pregnancy because they tempt you to ignore messages of tiredness from your body. The essence of caring for your pregnant self is getting 'in tune' with the rhythms of your body and becoming aware of your special needs. Nobody else can do this for you and the answers are not to be found in books. The ancient Greeks used to say 'Know yourself'. A feeling of wellbeing in pregnancy grows from this. •What do you most enjoy about your pregnancy? And what least?

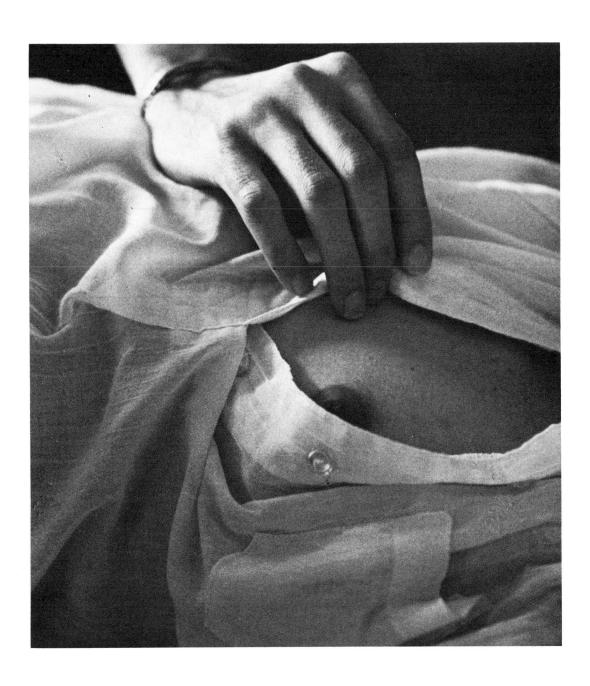

Seventeen Weeks

Reflections & Observations

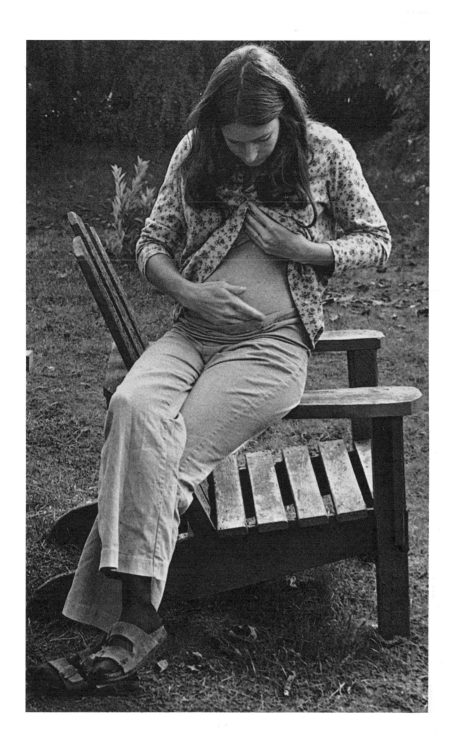

Eighteen Weeks

The baby moves. Some time during the last few weeks or very soon now you feel a sudden knock from inside you, or perhaps a flutter of movement as if butterflies were beating their wings. You wonder if it really can be the baby or if it is only your imagination. •You have felt *life*. Another being is nestled deep in your body, shielded from harm, floating in an inner sea, swimming and turning, twisting and sometimes somersaulting. The baby pushes with its feet against the springy walls of the uterus and so propels itself in all directions. If this is your first baby you may not notice these movements for another two weeks or so or even think they are caused by intestinal gas. Note down in your diary the date when you first feel movement as this can be useful in working out exactly when the baby is due. •There may have been times when you have thought of the baby as just a lump or a bump, or even as a sort of parasite. But it is clear now that it is a real baby. Another *person* is coming to being. •At this stage of pregnancy already twenty-five quarts of blood are flowing through the placenta to your baby every day.

Eighteen Weeks

Reflections & Observations

Nineteen Weeks

You may notice that you are dreaming more. Many women experience vivid fantasies about their bodies, the birth and the baby. Some have erotic dreams. Some dream in colour for the first time. •This is all part of a tuning in to your body, getting more deeply into your feelings, not just using your body like a tool, but living in it. •There isn't any way you *should* feel. All the emotions you have are the outcome of your personal experience and are valid. Let the feelings come, the good and the bad. Notice new sensations: the weight, shape and texture of your breasts, abdomen and vagina, the curve of bone, the swelling of flesh as you drift out of sleep. Enjoy the vitality that pours from the centre of your body and which gives birth to new images of lushness and succulence. Don't underestimate the importance of feelings. A positive sense of your body through the different phases of pregnancy may be as important for you and your baby as the right medical care. •Being aware of your body, especially the parts which cradle your baby and bring it to birth, is easiest when you are re-laxed. Relaxation is not only a passive 'letting go' but can be an active discovery of self. •When a muscle contracts it thickens and shortens. Rest the palm of your hand over the back of your neck. Now clench your jaw, grit your teeth and tense your neck. Notice what you feel under your hand. Then relax the muscles. Select other parts of your body, muscles in your arms and legs for example, and note what happens when they contract. The muscles tighten, go hard, and the bundles of fibre which make up the muscle get shorter. •Muscles respond automatically to strong emotions. Close your eyes and imagine lying in bed in a dark room about to drift off to sleep. Allow yourself a few minutes in which to feel comfortable and relaxed. Your breathing gets slower . . . Suddenly you hear the door opening slowly, creaking. What other sounds do you hear? Can you hear someone's step? Is someone there? Is it someone you love or a menacing presence? Notice what has happened to your breathing and which muscles have contracted. Then relax. •Can you think of any incident in your life when anger or fear has produced physical effects, for example, going to the dentist, taking an examination, having an interview, or doing something which you did not want discovered? Blood pressure can go up by as much as fifty points as a consequence of strong emotion. The constriction of muscles, the bronchi leading to and from the lungs and blood vessels can result in digestive and circulatory disturbance, changes in breathing, such as asthma, migraine and other stress headaches, and pain in the back, shoulders, and neck. In each case a message is being sent from the brain which results in contraction of the muscles concerned. •Even if you do not have aches and pains, when muscles are contracted unnecessarily energy is wasted, leaving you exhausted at the end of the day. Sometimes you may even be tired when getting up in the morning, because even in sleep one can be locked in tension. •Give a long breath out through your mouth, relax right down to your toes, and then just let the breath come in again through your nose. Go on breathing like this and relax more with each breath out. Think of the breath out and the breath in will look after itself. Sit or lie listening to the sound of your own slow breathing. Relax completely and try to let a pleasurable awareness of your own body fill your consciousness. Now think of your shoulder girdle and explore the capacity for movement in your shoulders, first one at a time and then both together. Draw circles with them, moving in all directions very slowly and smoothly. Release of the shoulders is essential for easy breathing, and this applies whether you are breathing deeply or shallowly in labour and however slow or fast you want to breathe. Let your shoulders settle comfortably into their natural position. Then draw them down, pulling them towards your feet so that your neck feels longer. Hold this position for a few seconds and then let the tension go. Your shoulders will feel relaxed and loose. This is how they should be right through labour. Consciously release your shoulders in this way whenever you confront a challenge or feel under stress. •What images and ideas help you relax best?

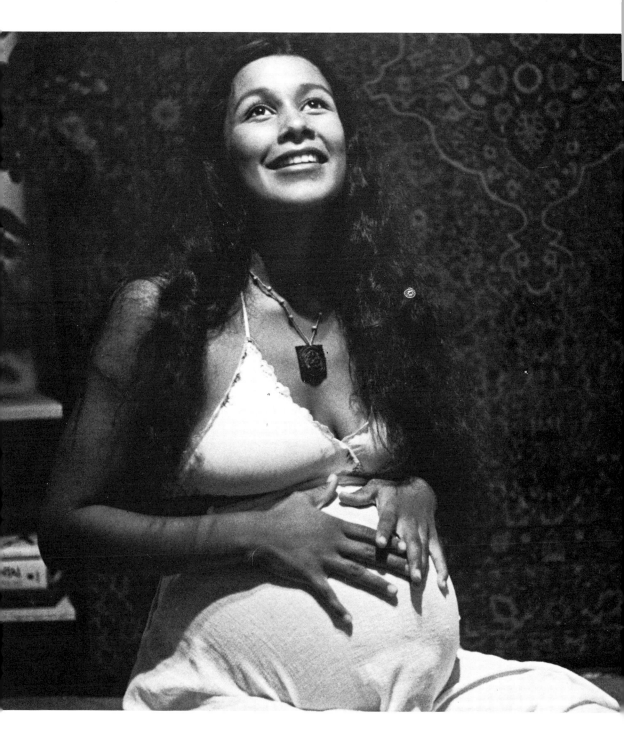

Nineteen Weeks

Reflections & Observations

Twenty Weeks

When you practice relaxation try some upright resting postures, because when you are in labour it is useful to be able to relax in positions in which your pelvis is wide and in which gravity helps your baby to press down through the cervix. •The labouring woman in the photograph is sitting up with her husband, who is sitting in front of her, supporting the small of her back with a firm hand, while another helper is gently massaging any residual tension out of her shoulder. Give a long breath out and release completely. Continue to breathe slowly and completely and feel your body open. Listen to the sound of your own breathing and with each breath out relax more deeply. •Experiment with similar relaxation while crouching, putting a pillow on the headboard of the bed and kneeling with arms and head on the pillow, or kneeling on a beanbag. See how it feels when you are in an all-fours position on the beanbag too. In these positions you tip the baby forward away from your spine, so they are good postures if you have backache in labour. They also make it easy for your partner to massage your back. Some women enjoy being massaged, stroked or held during labour. It is a good idea to start with a shoulder massage, and perhaps massage of the inner thighs, buttocks and feet too, in pregnancy, so that you get to know what helps you relax best. When you are actually in labour you may not want the same kind of massage, you may want it in different places, or you may not want it at all. But it will have been useful anyway to help the easing of tension during pregnancy. •The baby weighs about 0.45 kg. now and becomes more and more active. It is about 25 cm., half its length at birth. Every baby has its own patterns of waking and sleeping. When the baby wakes up, it moves vigorously and may even flip right over.

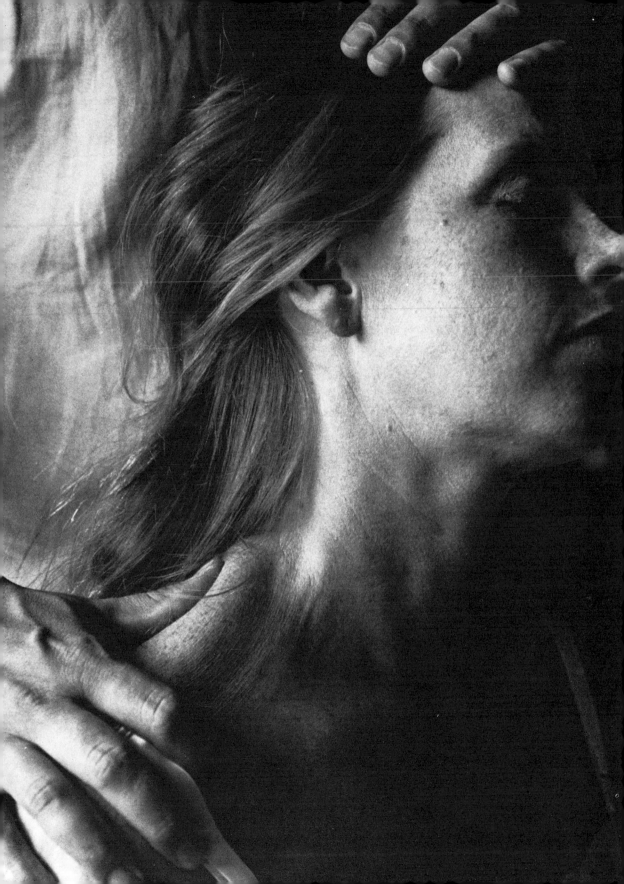

Twenty Weeks

Reflections & Observations

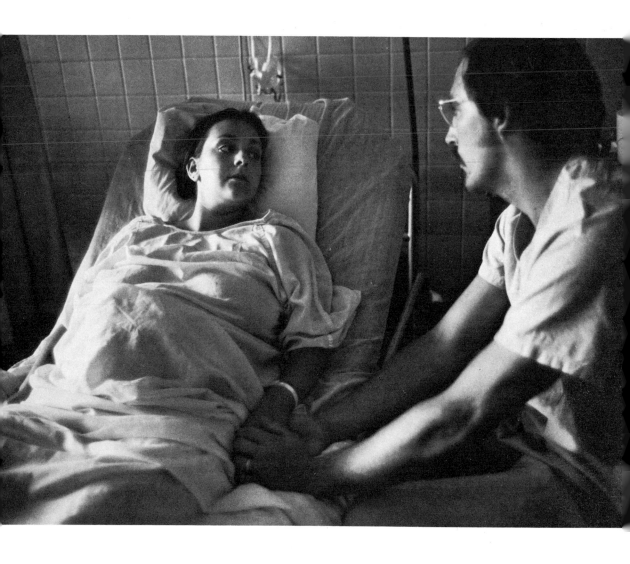

Twenty-one Weeks

If you have not done so before, now is a good time to start talking with your partner about his feelings about the coming baby, the birth and the changes that are bound to come into your life as a couple. •In the past men often tried not to get involved. Having a baby, and caring for it afterwards, was entirely women's business. Men who were present in childbirth were considered odd. Today men enjoy sharing the experience and helping their partners not only with their breathing and relaxation and by massage and so on, but also just by being there and giving their love. •The most important way of sharing is giving emotional support rather than directing a technical performance. This is sometimes forgotten or considered less helpful than timing contractions with a stop-watch or beating time with a finger so that the woman breathes evenly. Such practices can sometimes superimpose a kind of mechanical 'physical jerks' on the spontaneous rhythms of the woman's body and turn labour into a battle between the correct exercises and her natural feelings. •You can start now by experimenting with ways in which he can convey loving support. When you are both in bed have a short practice session. You close your eyes and relax. Then *through touch alone* he explores ways in which he can communicate confidence, trust, love and understanding. Tell him what feels good and when the non-verbal message gets through to you clearly. Discuss it together and then explore some different kinds of touch on other parts of your body and see whether they are more effective. •A man can be strong and still tender, a success in his job and yet capable of responding with love and understanding to a baby's needs. Sharing in childbirth has added a new dimension to fatherhood.

Twenty-one Weeks

Reflections & Observations

Twenty-two Weeks

The walls of the uterus have an enormous capacity to stretch. Each bundle of muscle fibres can expand up to forty times its usual length. In pregnancy the uterus both stretches and grows, forming new muscle. •Your skin is stretched from underneath and may develop silvery marks which will fade away after birth but never quite disappear. Massage with an oil or cream to keep the skin supple may help reduce this. The parts where stretch marks are most likely to occur are your abdomen, buttocks and breasts. Your partner can help by stroking in oil each night. •At about this stage of pregnancy it is useful to start practicing *Touch Relaxation* together. The idea is that you tense up the muscles of one part of your body and then your partner rests his hands on the part that feels tightened. As soon as you feel the warmth and weight of his touch you release, as if flowing out towards his touch. In this way he can give you non-verbal signals to relax which is much easier than being *told* to relax when you're feeling tense. He should touch you slowly and firmly, and keep his hands in place until he has felt all the tension flow out. Try this on the front of the shoulders, which are very important, the inside upper arm, the inside thighs, the back of your neck, your forehead and your feet. (When your partner touches your feet he should do so very firmly or it will tickle.) The same kind of touch relaxation can also be very helpful in labour. •From now on rehearse this once or twice a week and when you get within six weeks of the birth practice a little every day if possible.

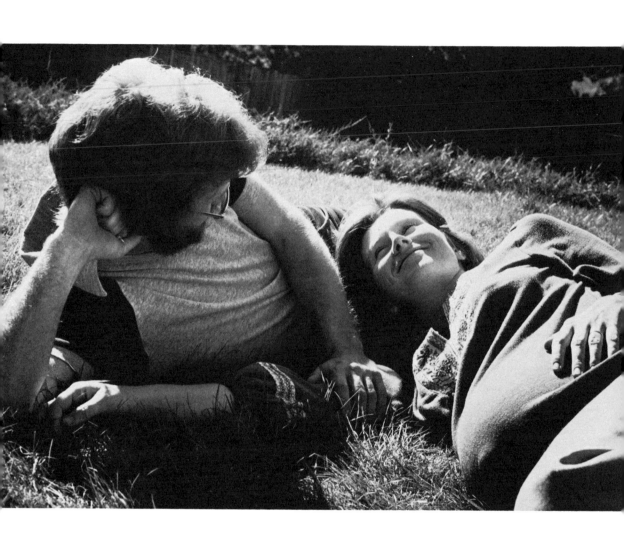

Twenty-two Weeks

Reflections & Observations

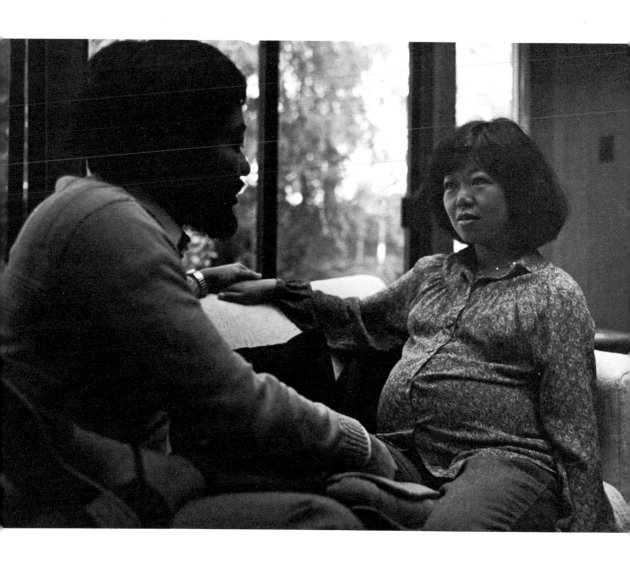

Twenty-three Weeks

Most labours are painful at some phase, especially just before the uterus is completely open towards the end of the first stage. This pain is quite different from the pain of injury. It is 'pain with a purpose', the pain of working muscles and stretching tissues. •The opening of the cervix is estimated in centimetres. At ten centimetres the way is open for the baby to be pressed down through the birth canal and be born. Between six centimetres and full dilatation contractions often hurt, at least when they are at their tightest, usually about halfway through each one. So it makes sense to have techniques to handle pain. In childbirth education classes you can learn breathing and relaxation skills. But even then the information sometimes stays 'all in the head' and it helps to rehearse contractions with a stimulus that really is quite uncomfortable or even painful. To simulate contractions your partner can pinch a little flesh on your inside thigh, gradually squeezing tighter and tighter until after about fifteen seconds he is pinching hard. He retains his grip for another fifteen to twenty seconds and then slowly releases it. The whole rehearsed contraction should last between one and two minutes. As the contraction starts give a long breath out through your mouth, the welcoming breath. Use regular rhythmic breathing to 'go with' your contraction as it increases in strength, reaches its peak and then dies away. •You will probably find that steady eye contact with your partner helps and if he encourages you and lets you know you are doing well this is even better. The same applies when you are in labour. •When the contraction is over give a long breath out through your mouth – the 'resting' breath. •Even if you didn't manage well with a contraction, relax completely at the end of it, for if you are tense in between contractions you quickly get tired and they become much more painful. When you rehearse you can practice taking catnaps in between contractions, preparing yourself for using the interval between them for a complete letting go. •It also helps to think of the work that the uterus is doing, pulling open the cervix and pressing the baby down. Concentrate on the picture of the uterus opening and release your shoulders, arms, legs and abdominal wall. As each contraction starts think, 'Good, here's another one', and start working with it. •You have only one contraction at a time. Don't worry about the next one. Meet each as it comes and breathe your way through it. When it finishes think, 'Goodbye. That one will never come back again.' It is one step forward to having your baby in your arms. Practice these simulated contractions once or twice a week and when you get to six weeks before the birth rehearse some every day if you can.

Twenty-three Weeks

Reflections & Observations

Twenty-four Weeks

Have you thought how you would like to feed your baby? Breast milk is the best milk for human babies, cows' milk for calves. •One of the main problems with bottlefeeding is that the baby's intake of protein, sodium, potassium and calcium is much higher than for breast milk. If you are giving your baby cereals as well the concentration of salts is still higher. •In the first five months of life a baby's kidneys, which are still immature, can't easily adjust the fluid balance when fed such a diet and have difficulty excreting the very concentrated urine which is produced. •If a baby gets a stomach upset or gastro-enteritis with diarrhoea and vomiting a diet of artificial milk and solid foods tends to aggravate the illness. •But breastfeeding is more than just a way of giving your baby milk. It is a way of communicating through the touch of your two bodies. A baby at the breast is at just the right distance to focus on the mother's face and see the messages conveyed by her eyes and mouth, so that the two can begin to have conversations long before any words are used. •If you decide to bottlefeed your baby, it is very important to make up the feed correctly, to sterilize all equipment used, never to keep a bottle warm for later use and always to hold the baby close. •At this stage of pregnancy your baby is about 30 cm. long. Hair is growing on the head and eyebrows are finely etched. By now the baby inside you is very active and you may be able to distinguish between a kick from a foot, a knock from a hand and a movement from its bottom as it swings from side to side. When the baby is asleep it curls up in its own characteristic sleeping posture which varies with different babies. Your baby will probably sleep in this position once it is born.

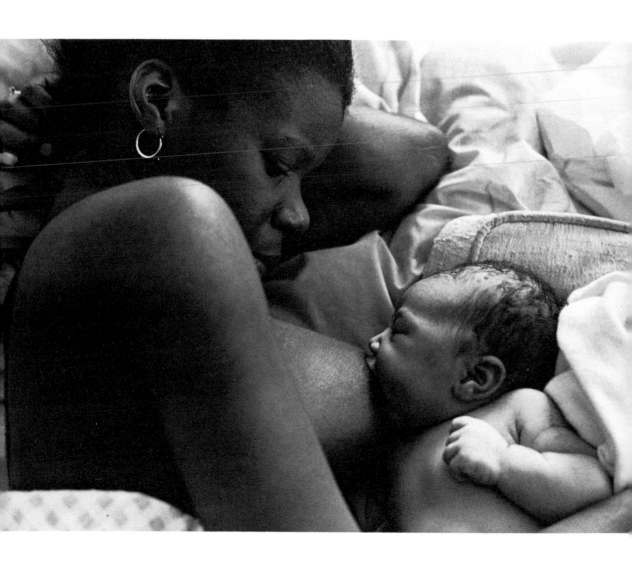

Twenty-four Weeks

Reflections & Observations

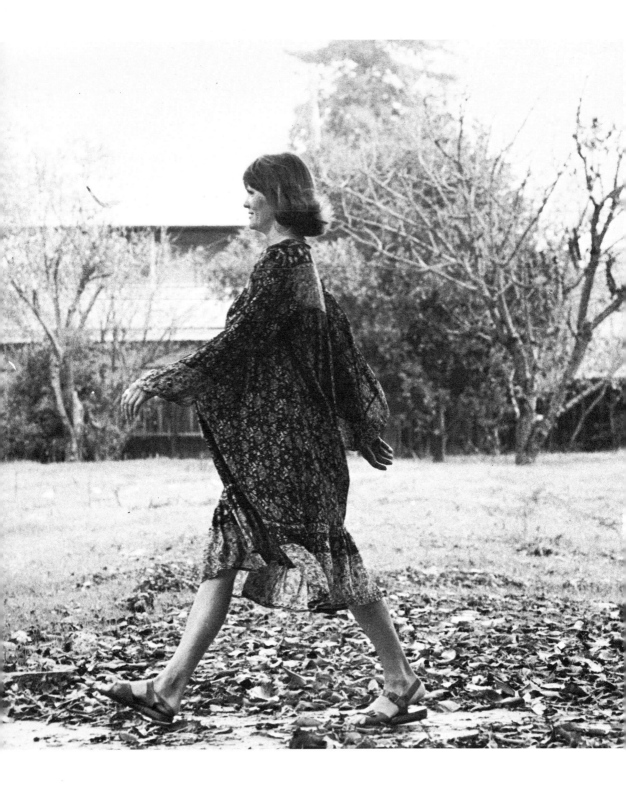

Twenty-five Weeks

Standing straight and tall helps to hold the baby in the cradle of the pelvis and avoids strain on your lower back and shoulders. Lift your rib cage (it happens automatically when you breathe in with a complete breath), tuck your tail in, and notice how this action firms the abdominal muscles and lifts the baby into your pelvis like an egg in an eggcup. •Feel as if an invisible rope is drawing the top of the centre of your head upward, and that the rope passes down through the middle of your body to the balls of your feet, pulling straight and firm. •As your tummy gets bigger the tendency is to hollow the lower back, roll back on the heels, let the arches of the feet drop and then, because in this position it is easy to lose your balance, to stick your bottom out and fling shoulders back to compensate for the change in the centre of gravity. The result is backache concentrated in the area where the pelvis joins the spine and also behind the shoulders. •As you pass a mirror or catch your reflection in the plate glass of an office or shop, notice how you are standing and take the opportunity of correcting any slumping and muscle slackness. •Use a wheeled shopping carrier and try to get help lifting a heavy box of groceries. If you must carry heavy weights hold them close to your body or distribute the load so that it is equally balanced on both sides. When moving furniture, cleaning out the bath or making a bed get down close to it by bending your knees and adopting a crouching or squatting position.

Twenty-five Weeks

Reflections & Observations

Twenty-six Weeks

It is often said that pregnant women are calm and placid, untroubled by things that normally disturb them. Perhaps this is true of some, but a great many others find themselves laughing and crying more readily and are deeply affected by everything happening around them: other people's joy and sorrow, the terrible things happening in the world – war and famine, cruelty, aggression and hate. •The expectant mother is not insulated from suffering. She knows she is bearing a child to live in the real world. It is not just a question of buying equipment for the baby, choosing tiny clothes and preparing for the birth, but the frightening responsibility of introducing another being into a world torn by violence. •You may find yourself especially vulnerable emotionally and readily distressed by TV documentaries or news in which human suffering – especially that of children – is vividly depicted. It seems to be part of a process of emotional change which prepares you *and* your partner for responding to the baby's needs with sensitivity and awareness. •Pregnancy is a time when both expectant parents often spontaneously re-assess their lives and for this reason it can be an unsettled period. It can help to bring this out into the open and discuss your goals and the values which hold most meaning for you. •There are things to consider too about the style of parenthood and the nature of your relationship as a couple as compared with those of friends, relatives and your own parents. Do you want to be the same kind of parents as your own mothers and fathers or different in any way?

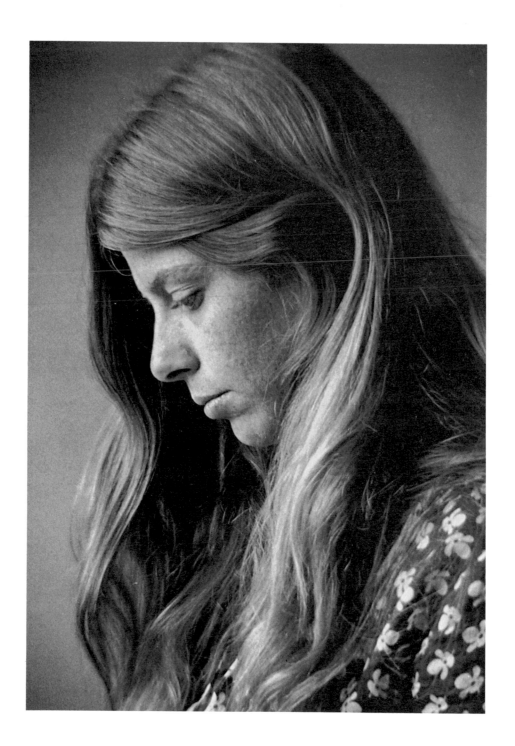

Twenty-six Weeks

Reflections & Observations

Twenty-seven Weeks

Have you thought how you want the birth to be for your baby? •As we have seen, all medications for pain relief pass through your bloodstream into the baby's bloodstream. Sometimes they only affect the baby slightly. Drugs like Pethidine make the baby drowsy, and often slow to suck and not very inclined to open its eyes. And used in high doses most anaesthetic drugs can make it difficult for a baby to breathe without help at birth. •You can learn yourself how to reduce pain by releasing muscle tension and letting your uterus work and your body give birth. Learn how to breathe *with* contractions instead of fighting them or trying to run from pain. This can help your baby as well as you. Contractions come in waves, following one another in sea rhythms, and when you ride the waves with a relaxed body and rhythmic breathing, your mind focuses on the creative work of the uterus. This is active birth-giving. •Practice first by resting on the bed or in a comfortable chair with your hands spread over the curve of your lower tummy. Breathe right down to where you can feel your hands pressing so that the wave of your breathing flows slowly through your body and your hands rise with the breath in and falls with the breath out. •Now sit on an upright chair facing the chair back, legs wide apart and leaning forward with your forearms on a cushion on the chair back. Your partner rests both hands firmly at either side of your spine at waist level. Breathe so that the main level of breathing awareness is where you feel the hand pressure, in through your nose and out through a relaxed mouth. This is deep chest breathing and it is useful during contractions. •When you feel that this breathing comes easily he raises his hands so that he is pressing on the lower part of your shoulder blades. Change your breathing so that it is quicker and lighter and the main level of breathing activity is where you feel the pressure. You may like to do this in and out through your mouth. Keep it very light. It sometimes helps to think of a seagull's wings in flight as they sweep up and down. For this reason I call it 'seagull breathing'. •When contractions get powerful you will probably want to lift your breathing higher and to slightly increase the rate and use this seagull breathing over the tops of the contractions. Towards the end of the first stage of labour contractions get fast and furious. They last one minute or more and the interval between them may be less than a minute. It is helpful to have a still shallower and quicker kind of breathing to handle these contractions. To practice, rest your fingertips against your cheeks, plumping the cheeks under your fingers so that you are smiling slightly. Release your mouth, drop your head slightly forward and release your throat muscles. Now breathe very lightly in and out through parted lips, at first like a steam train heard in the distance, chugging slowly up hill. You can stress one breath out of every three or four if it helps you establish a steady rhythm. Now let your little train speed up as it reaches level ground. Make sure that your shoulders and neck muscles are completely released as you do this or you will start to gasp and the breathing will get heavier. This then leads to over-breathing and hyperventilation. If at any time you lose the rhythm or find you are getting tense, do a crisp blow out through pursed lips, allow a quick breath in to follow, and carry on with the quick, light effortless breathing. Once you are comfortable with this you may not need to emphasize any one breath. It then becomes a rapid, even breathing rhythm rather like the movement of a humming-bird's wings as it flutters poised in front of a flower or like the light beat of a butterfly's wings. So you may like to think of it as 'humming-bird' or 'butterfly' breathing.

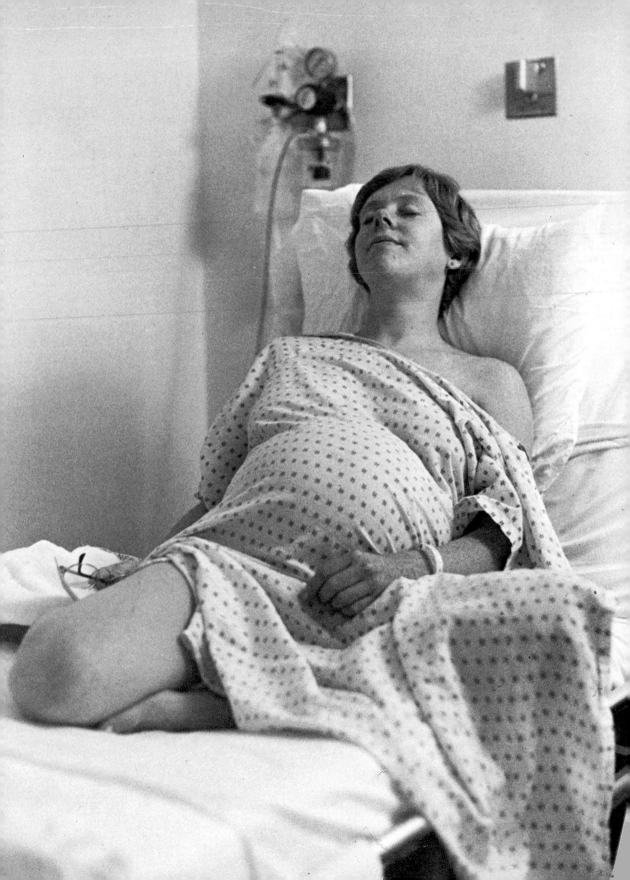

Twenty-seven Weeks

Reflections & Observations

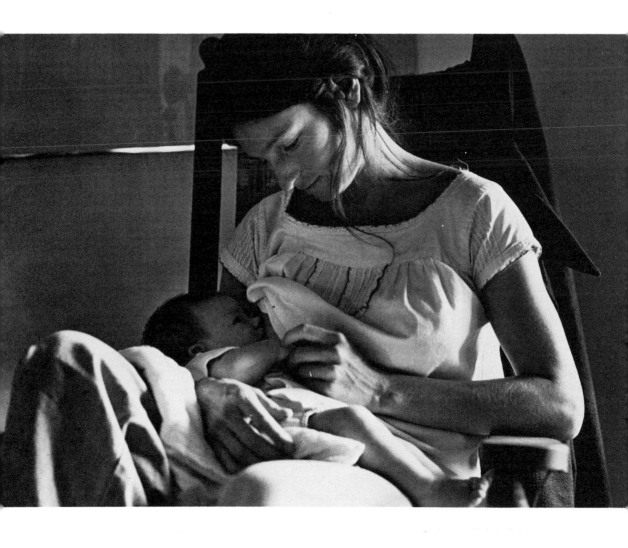

Twenty-eight Weeks

When you think of your baby, how do you imagine it? Sleeping and beautiful or red with rage and screaming its head off? When you think of the future how do you imagine it will be to have a baby in the house? •Dream and reality are sometimes very far apart, especially for a woman whose partner does not share willingly in at least some of the new and formidable tasks of parenthood. The sheer amount of work a baby makes can hardly be believed. At first each feed may take as long as an hour, because many babies suck, fall asleep and then wake to nuzzle again. Remember, though, that the baby gets most of the milk in the first 5 – 10 minutes. So small, frequent feeds are better than long ones in which you try to fill up the baby. A tiny baby's stomach is small and you cannot stoke it up sure that the baby will last out for four hours. In fact, many new babies feed at very irregular intervals in the first weeks, and some seem to be sucking all the time. The baby will not want the same quantity of milk at every feed, any more than an adult eats the same sized meals right through the day or on each day of the week. Be guided by your baby and you cannot go wrong. •It's difficult to prepare for the feelings of inadequacy and guilt that most of us encounter from time to time as mothers. Sharing can help. Everything seems much worse when you think you are the only person to feel like this. You are not alone. It is all part of the 'growing pains' of parenthood. •This is the time when your baby's brain is having a developmental spurt. The part involved with thinking, the cerebral cortex, is growing fast. The little creature in there is a fully intelligent, distinct being, with the foundations of later personality already established.

Twenty-eight Weeks

Reflections & Observations

Twenty-nine Weeks

How is the baby to be welcomed? With loud noises and rough handling or with gentleness and in peace, and with consideration for its sensitive nervous system which is just encountering the stimuli of the world around? •The new-born child is a traveller in time who has just taken the first step over the threshold of life. The baby is not just a product of a birth, but a unique person. •Loving arms wait to hold the child. The parents' faces greet their baby in exultation and then soothe her, telling her that after all the world is not such a bad place. Lights can be dimmed so that the baby opens its eyes and the gaze of the newborn meets shadow, glimmer, half light, and above all a smiling human face. •The child feels the warm closeness of contact with the mother, and having left her body returns to it to be held in the arms and to suck at her breast. •Some time around now the baby inside you tips head down in the uterus. The head is the largest part and fits snugly into the lower segment of the uterus. The baby probably helps this by its kicking. He or she steps against the bouncing muscular wall of the uterus with a reflex stepping movement which it demon-strates also after birth, so somersaulting itself over and then, because by now it is a tight fit, the head becomes fixed in the lower segment.

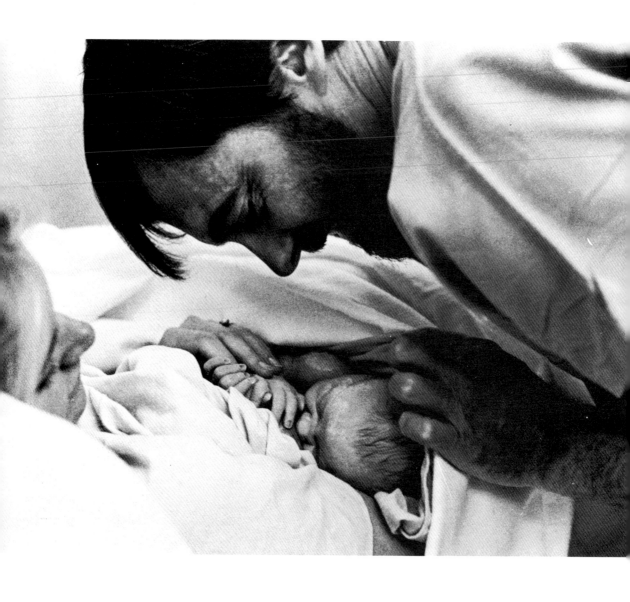

Twenty-nine Weeks

Reflections & Observations

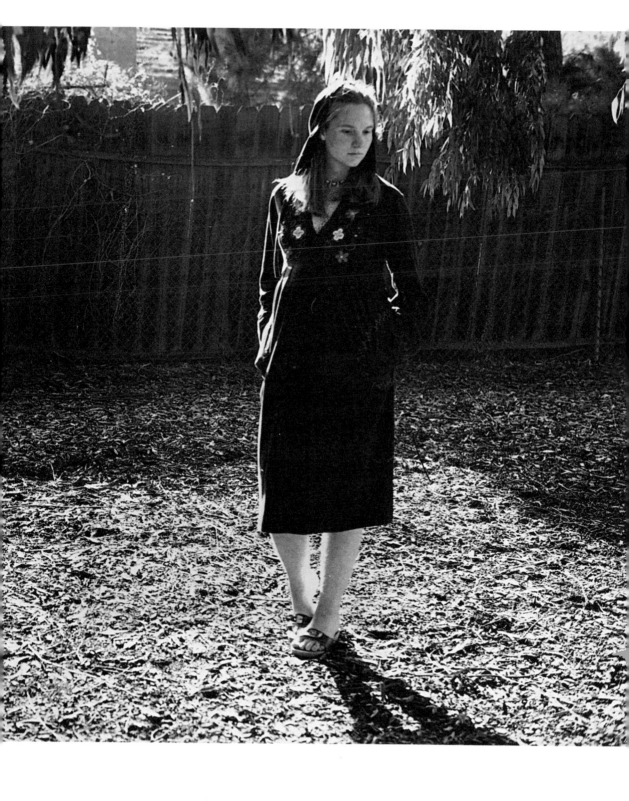

Thirty Weeks

Now the life of the mind sometimes seems to exist independently of everything that is going on outside the body and surges with all the feelings aroused by the baby inside, the pressure, the tightenings of the uterus and the blood pulsing through the pelvic organs. You find yourself waiting for the baby's movements, however faint, and it is hard to concentrate on the external world. For many women it is as if they are having a two-way conversation, one with the world outside and the people round about and the other with the baby inside them. Now and then you may find it difficult to concentrate on activities in the 'real' world because of your baby's presence. This is one important way in which you are becoming ready for being aware of and responsive to your baby *after* birth. •Some forgetfulness, a more relaxed attitude to time, not minding so much when plans don't work out as they should, lack of concern about all the petty inessentials which usually cause worry are characteristic of this stage of pregnancy. A pregnant woman has a new perspective. Perhaps for the first time she has life in its *right* perspective.

Thirty Weeks

Reflections & Observations

Thirty-one Weeks

You can also use some of the images of Yoga to 'centre down' further into your body. Give a long breath out through a soft, relaxed mouth and feel as if the breath were flowing completely out from your body at its core, as if it were pouring from your navel, till the tide turns and you breathe in through your nose, drawing fresh air into your body as if through your navel. Let the air flood in and fill you with its life-giving energy, suffuse and bathe your whole body as if with light. •Become more aware of the flow of your breathing, listening to it in stillness, letting it take its own time, not forcing it. Imagine the air you breathe is golden light and open yourself to it so that it pours into every part of you. Then imagine it is cool, green light. See in your mind different colours – violet, brown, white, dove grey, blue – and notice the sensations aroused in different parts of your body. •It is better not to start doing Yoga positions which are strenuous or painful now, but if you are already accustomed to doing Yoga carry on with it, using the wall or a chair to help you keep your balance if necessary, and simply omitting any postures in which you are forced to hold your breath, as well as those which involve lying flat on your back.

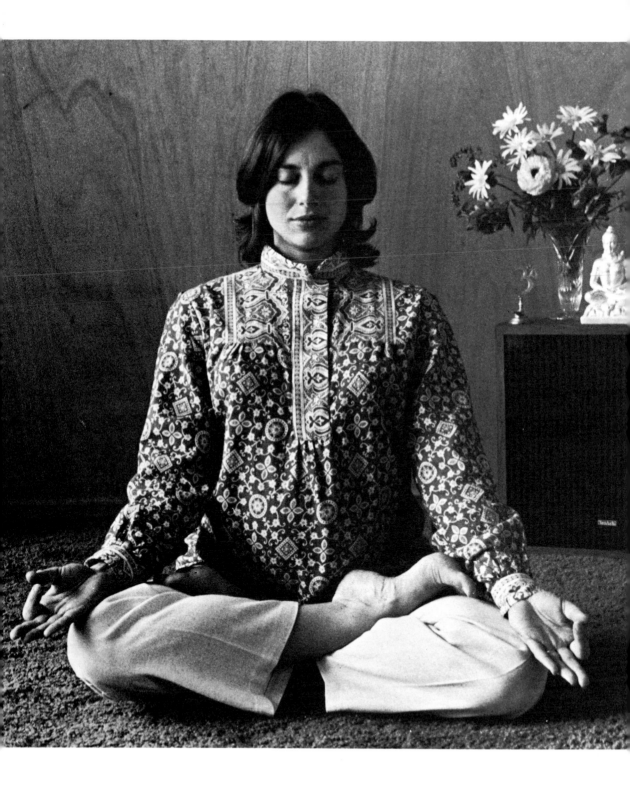

Thirty-one Weeks

Reflections & Observations

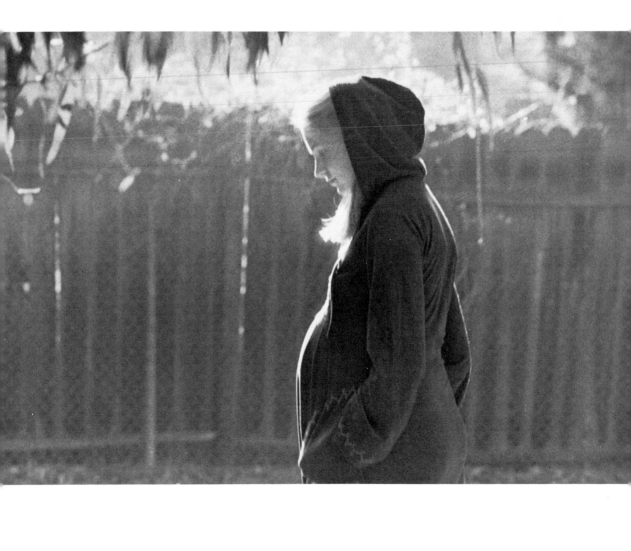

Thirty-two Weeks

At about this stage of pregnancy previously unacknowledged fear may flood into you, especially in the middle of the night. Fear is readily passed from one person to another. It is communicated through smell and unconscious body language – changes in the depth and rate of breathing, tightening and twitching of muscles, through skin changes (gooseflesh, for example), changes in facial expression, gesture and the way we stand and move. Fear also changes body chemistry. The whole metabolism adapts to cope with the threat. •Since nutrients, oxygen and other chemicals in the mother's blood filter through the placenta into the baby's bloodstream it is highly likely that powerful emotions can affect your baby. •This used to be considered an 'old wives' tale' (why old *wives*? – don't old men have any tales to tell too?). Though it is not true that lifting your arms above your head to hang the washing can twist the cord round the baby's neck, or that wanting strawberries and not having them gives the baby a strawberry mark (both myths of this kind), there was an element of truth in the tales which stressed the importance of a tranquil mind and happy relationships. Perhaps we had too much faith in the 'scientific' way and failed to understand those things women knew and passed down one to another. •If you experience strong negative emotions of any kind, take time to think through why you are feeling so and let positive emotions flow out instead. Fear is there to be met and worked with. Acknowledge it and then allow positive feelings to well up in place of fear. •Anxiety can interfere with sleep, and many pregnant women who wake up because they need to empty their bladders or the baby is kicking vigorously then lie awake worrying. It doesn't matter that you are not asleep, provided that you are relaxed. Worrying about not sleeping does far more harm than lying awake. Use this time to practice relaxation and rhythmic breathing, get up and do some restful, rather boring task or read or sew. As you do so, you may discover that fears of which you were not consciously aware come to the surface so that you can examine them, put them in perspective, work out practical ways of handling them and begin to think creatively instead.

Thirty-two Weeks

Reflections & Observations

Thirty-three Weeks

In some cultures they say that tender lovemaking during pregnancy 'nourishes' the baby. Some couples do not enjoy having intercourse any more once this stage of pregnancy is reached. Others enjoy it but usually want to experiment with different positions for comfort. Try intercourse with your partner behind you. You can either kneel forward, be on all fours, or lie on your side with your knees drawn up. Whatever position you choose, use pillows under your breasts or tummy for more comfort. Orgasm sometimes stimulates uterine contractions which continue after lovemaking and which can be worrying because you wonder if you are going into premature labour. •If you don't feel you want orgasm, tender stroking can be intensely pleasurable and help you to relax deeply. Some women feel they do not need orgasm at this stage of pregnancy and may even be a little frightened of it, but loving contact is important. Tell your partner where you want to be touched, and how, and guide his hand if necessary. •Notice how your body is when you are luxuriously relaxed like this. Notice your breathing, the way your whole weight sinks into the bed and pillows and spreads as if the body is flowing out from its boundaries. This is the relaxation you will need also for labour. •In the last weeks sex can be cumbersome. Just turning over in bed may be a major undertaking. Your uterus is 20 times heavier than before you became pregnant. You may feel there is no room inside for your partner's erect penis. When the baby has engaged (dropped into your pelvis) its head may feel like a heavy coconut in your vagina. Sometimes ejaculation causes a softening of the cervix with slight bleeding. If this happens your partner can use a condom so that the prostaglandin in semen is not deposited against your cervix. Then may be the time for pleasures without intercourse, each partner using hands and mouth to delight and satisfy the other. •Your baby has been responding to sound for some time. It can hear the regular thudding of your heart, loud noises outside, and the gurgling, pulsing, rumbling sounds of your digestive system. You may notice that the baby jumps around if you are at a concert. If you have a sonar scan the high-pitched sound, inaudible to our ears, will stir the baby into activity.

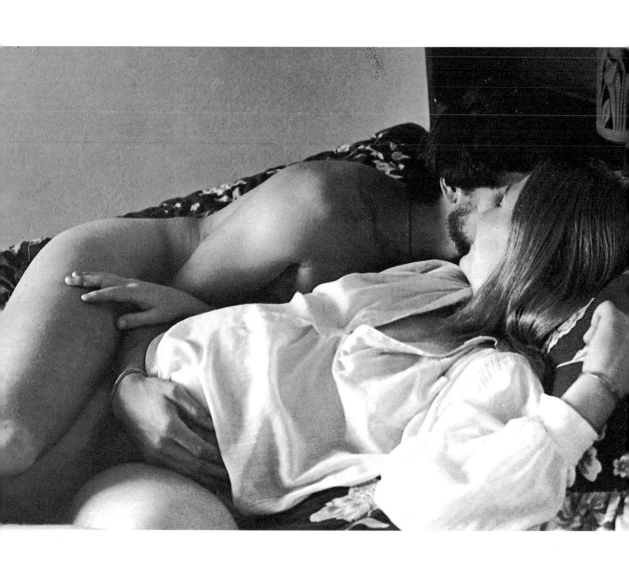

Thirty-three Weeks

Reflections & Observations

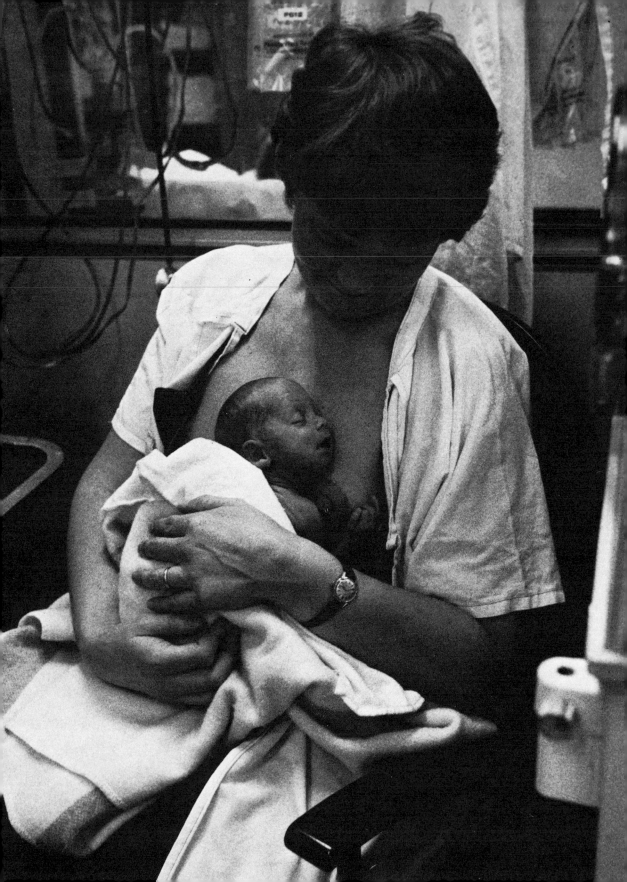

Thirty-four Weeks

The baby who is born this early needs specialized care. Birth should take place in a hospital with an intensive care unit where sophisticated, modern equipment and trained personnel are available to help your baby. •If your baby is in an intensive-care nursery it needs handling and loving just like any other baby, even though at first it may be lobster red and skinny and have adhesive tape, tubes and other appliances all over its little body. •Visit the nursery as often as possible and if your baby is in an incubator stroke and hold the little arms and legs through the cuffs in the plastic box. •You can express your own milk which can be fed to the baby even when it is still much too hard work for it to suck at your breast. You may like to help give the tube feeds and will quickly learn how to help the nurses care for your tiny baby. •When it is well enough to be lifted out, spend time holding, cuddling and talking to your child. During this month fat begins to develop underneath your baby's skin while it is still inside you and the wrinkles are gradually plumped out. •At this stage the baby's genitals are fully developed. The baby girl has inner and outer lips to her vagina and a tiny clitoris and the baby boy has a scrotum and a penis which can already become erect. The testes have usually descended by this time too, though often one or the other does not go down till after birth.

Thirty-four Weeks

Reflections & Observations

Thirty-five Weeks

It's about time you thought about the things you need for labour. If you are going into hospital you may like to pack your bag with a selection of comfort aids. If you are having your baby at home you'll need some of these things too:

- Two small cosmetic or artist's sponges (natural ones are best) for moistening your mouth and patting iced water on your face.
- A wide-mouthed vacuum flask to be stocked at the last moment with ice cubes or chips, for sucking between contractions.
- Toilet bag.
- Hairbrush, comb, ribbons if you have long hair.
- Talcum powder (unscented or lightly perfumed) and an oil or lotion for massage.
- Small aerosol or garden spray to be filled with ice-cold water for refreshing your face.
- Eau de cologne (not musky; plain bath cologne is best).
- Moisturized paper towels.
- Toothpaste and brush.
- Soap, washcloth.
- Deodorant.
- Vaseline, chapstick or lip gloss for dry lips.
- A picnic freeze pack or ice bag in case you want a cold compress.
- A hot water bottle.
- A neck cushion, either a small pillow or a Chinese dumb-bell shaped cushion to support your head comfortably forward.
- A rolling pin for ironing away backache.
- Small extra inflatable pillow or beach cushion for under knees or in small of back in case pillows are in short supply.
- Warm socks in case you feel cold.
- Short cotton nightdress if the hospital lets you wear your own.
- Some sustenance for your partner during labour and perhaps for you too.
- Playing cards, Scrabble, chess, crosswords or jigsaw puzzles, not too intellectually demanding.
- Books which can be enjoyed in short hops; poetry or humour, perhaps.
- Notebook, book for labour log, ballpoints.
- Painting, poster, photograph, computer drawing or the like for focal shape if you want to concentrate on something visual during contractions.
- Change for phone calls; list of numbers.
- Ear plugs, just in case labour is slow and gentle and you find noises of others in ward disturbing (useful for sleeping afterward too).

You may not use all of these things but they are useful to have. Let your partner know exactly what is in your bag and how each thing can be used, so that he isn't grappling in its depths as you are in the middle of a big contraction.

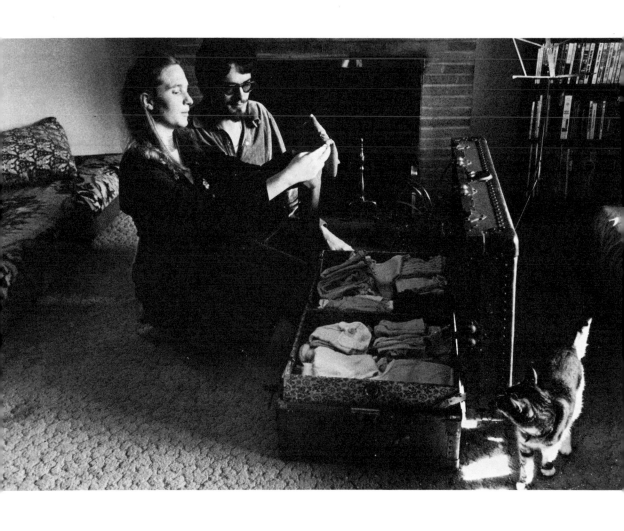

Thirty-five Weeks

Reflections & Observations

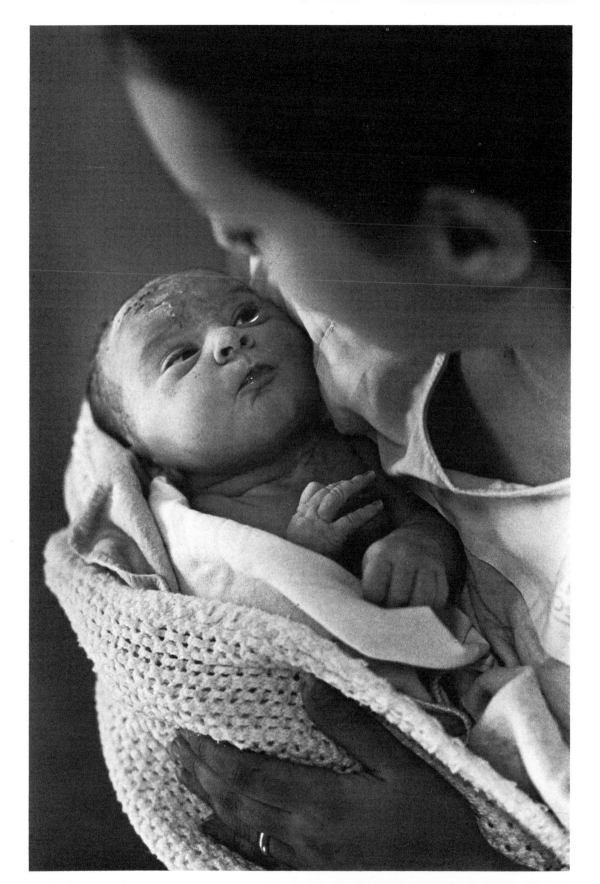

Thirty-six Weeks

The baby inside you will soon be outside. Incredible to think that after those long months of preparation and waiting the partnership is to be abruptly and dramatically changed, your baby pushed out into the world and at last a separate being in your arms. ●It's easy to think of the baby as just a part of the mother's body which has to be amputated, and some people approach birth with fear, as if it were a surgical operation rather than a natural physical process. Yet your body is beautifully designed for giving birth and the baby born at the right time is equipped with all the reflexes and skills to meet the challenge of life. ●The baby is its own self, a unique human being whom you will get to know and learn to understand. The answers are not to be found in books, but can only be learned from the child itself, the movements of the mouth and hands and whole body, the crying and peaceful sucking. Your baby will help you learn how to be a good mother. ●You may have decided that you will put your baby to the breast immediately after delivery. Give it time to begin to seek the nipple. When first given the breast most babies lick and sample before actually latching on to it and this licking and experimenting stimulates the nipple to become erect and the right shape for the baby.

Thirty-six Weeks

Reflections & Observations

Thirty-seven Weeks

Huge and melon-shaped, the curving bowl of your pregnant abdomen is stretched full with the baby, the enlarged uterus, heavy and ripe, the life-giving tree of blood vessels in the placenta and the great sac of water contained in the membranes. •You can reach down and feel your baby and its outlines under your hands. Wait till you feel a kick and notice the hard knobs of the little feet. By this time they may be under your ribs on the left or right side. •Follow the legs round to the firm curve of the buttocks and the solid trunk of the baby's body. Move down to the head, which may have already dipped down below your pubic bone so that you can feel only the shoulders at the very base of your tummy. •You may notice strange twinges, like small electric shocks, a kind of buzzing inside your vagina as the baby bounces its head against the hammock of pelvic muscles, using it like a trampoline. •Show your partner how he too can feel the different parts of your body. Parents and baby are beginning to get to know each other. •Your baby may get hiccups sometimes and you feel a quick knock—knock—knock or it may be turning its head quickly from side to side trying to find a lost thumb which it was happily sucking. Its heart beats at about double the rate of your own, at 120 to 160 beats a minute. Now your partner may even be able to hear this simply by resting his head against your abdomen.

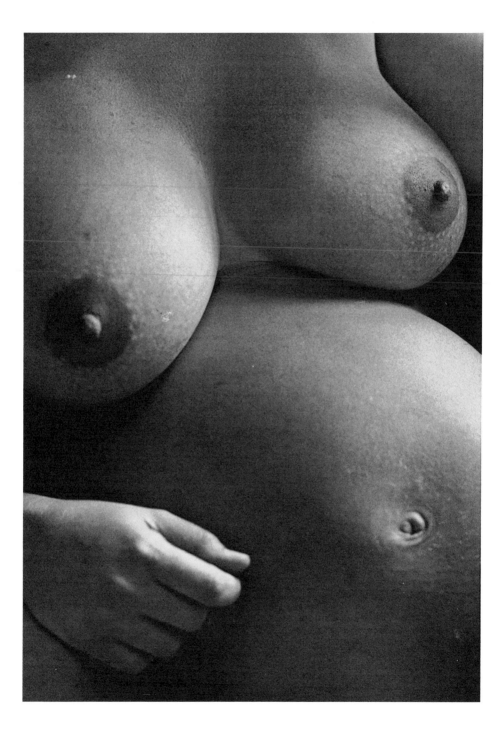

Thirty-seven Weeks

Reflections & Observations

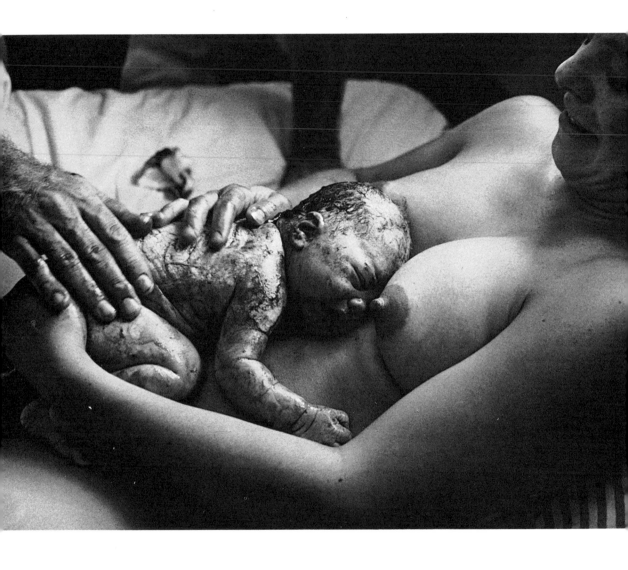

Thirty-eight Weeks

New babies do not look beautiful to everyone. But they are usually gorgeous to those mothers who give birth in an environment where they feel free to reach out and hold them in their arms immediately, with no cloth separating their two bodies. •Do not expect to fall in love with your baby right away. Loving a baby is like any love affair. Sometimes it is a sudden and overpowering feeling. At other times love dawns slowly. Sometimes you do not even know that you love until something happens that threatens to separate the two of you. •It helps to feel you belong together if you handle your baby often and care for it yourself. And just as this is an important part of growing into being a mother, so it can be for the man who is becoming a father too. From the first moments after delivery both of you can get to know your baby. •The baby has probably engaged in your pelvis by now, though sometimes this does not happen until you are in labour. If it has already occurred a week or two before, it does not mean that you are likely to go into a premature labour. By the end of pregnancy 300 quarts of blood a day are being pumped to your baby through the placenta. It takes only half a minute for blood to flow from the placenta to the baby and back to the placenta again. When you stand up your baby lies in your uterus as in a hammock, but when you lie down on your back the baby shifts position, perhaps because your spine is in the way, and starts to move over to one side or the other. You may notice that when you go to bed it is especially active and seems to wake up when you are ready to go to sleep.

Thirty-eight Weeks

Reflections & Observations

Thirty-nine Weeks

Around this time many women experience rhythmic, regular and gradually intensifying contractions of the uterus which make them think that labour must have started. But it is more like a rehearsal of labour and after several hours the contractions fade away. This is called sometimes 'false labour'. •If this happens you will probably feel very disappointed and may find that your morale drops. But contractions like this have usually done good preparatory work. They have moved the baby's presenting part – usually the head – down against your cervix and have started to pull up (efface) and open (dilate) the cervix. So it is not wasted. •The important thing is to avoid concentrating all your attention on pre-labour or early labour contractions. If contractions like this are tiring or irritating, try doing something entirely different. If you were lying in bed, get up and go for a brisk walk. If you were doing housework, have a relaxing bath, go to bed and sleep for a while. •You may be feeling some 'stage fright' now. The great day is about to dawn and you wonder whether you are well enough prepared, and after the impatience you probably felt in the last few weeks now think you are not 'ready.' It seems that you have been pregnant forever; you can't imagine not being pregnant. There seems to be a great gulf between the way you are now, heavy with child, and the 'afterwards.' It entails an enormous effort of the imagination to cast your mind forward into what it will be like after the baby comes. You want the baby out and yet you do not feel ready to surrender it yet. These conflicting emotions are characteristic of the last few weeks before the birth.

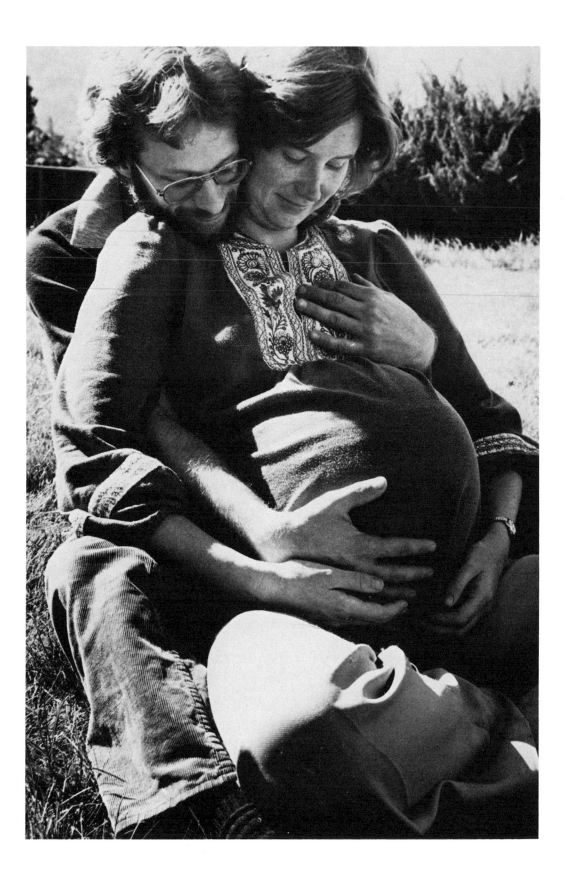

Thirty-nine Weeks

Reflections & Observations

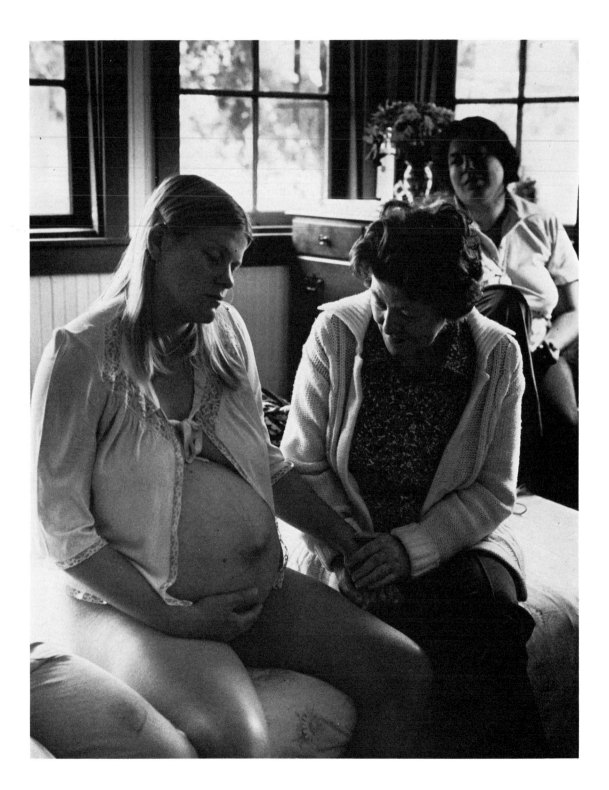

Forty Weeks

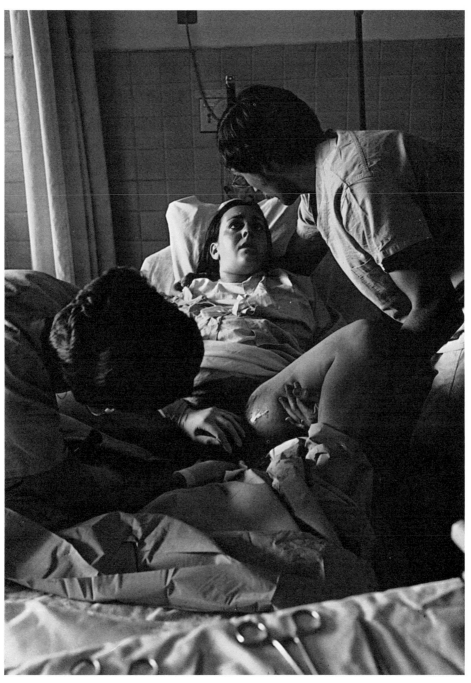

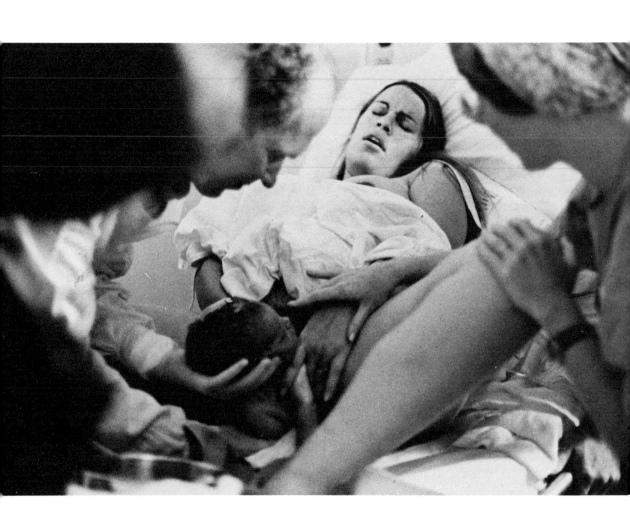

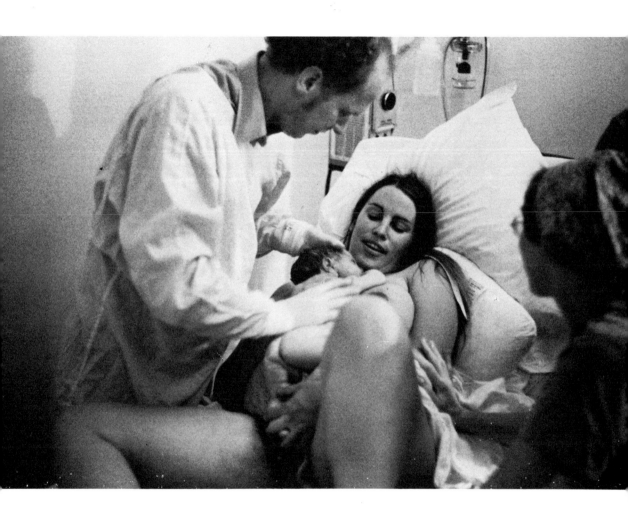

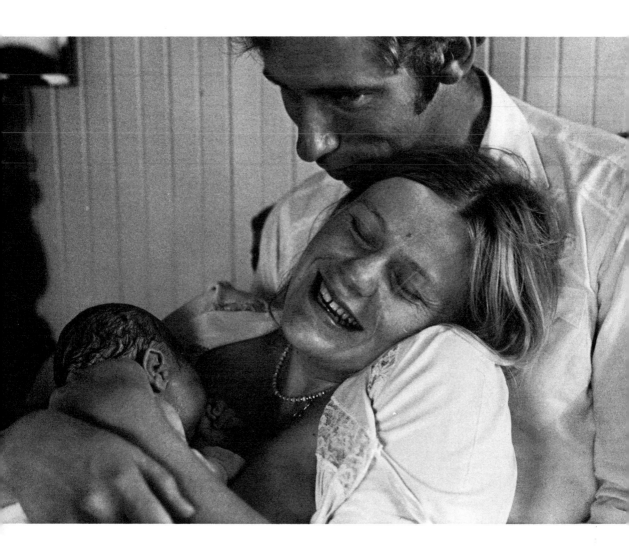

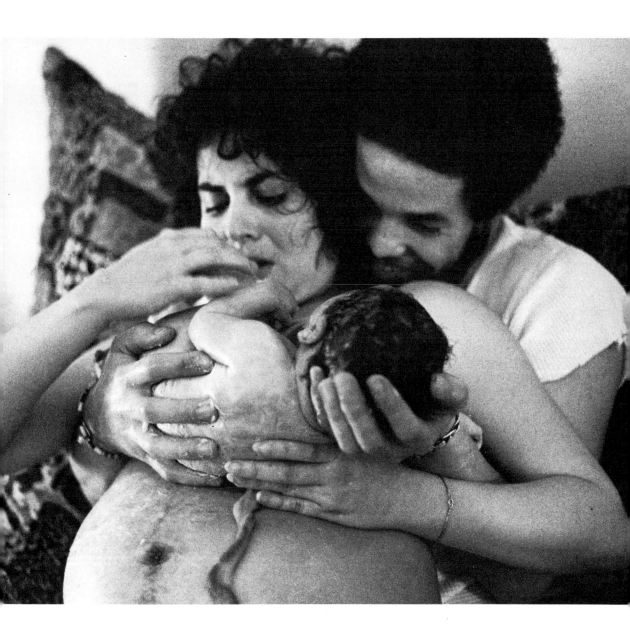

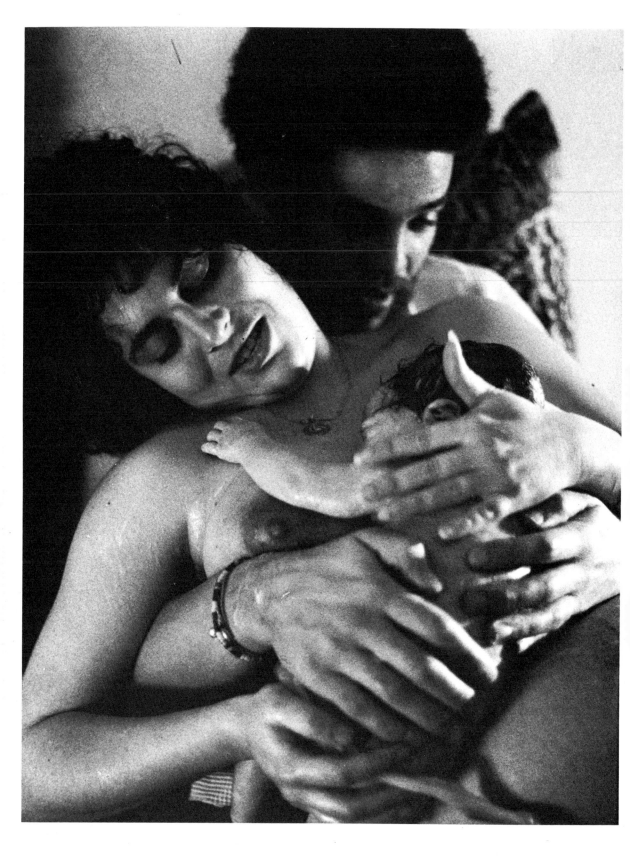

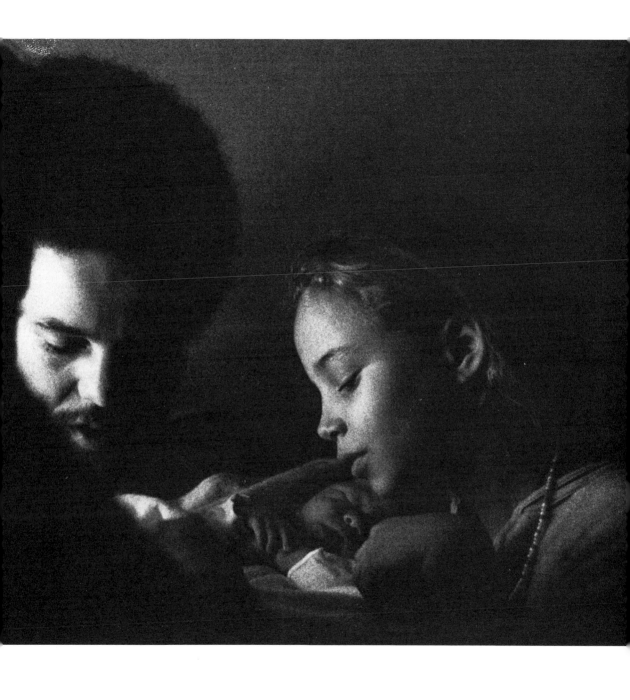

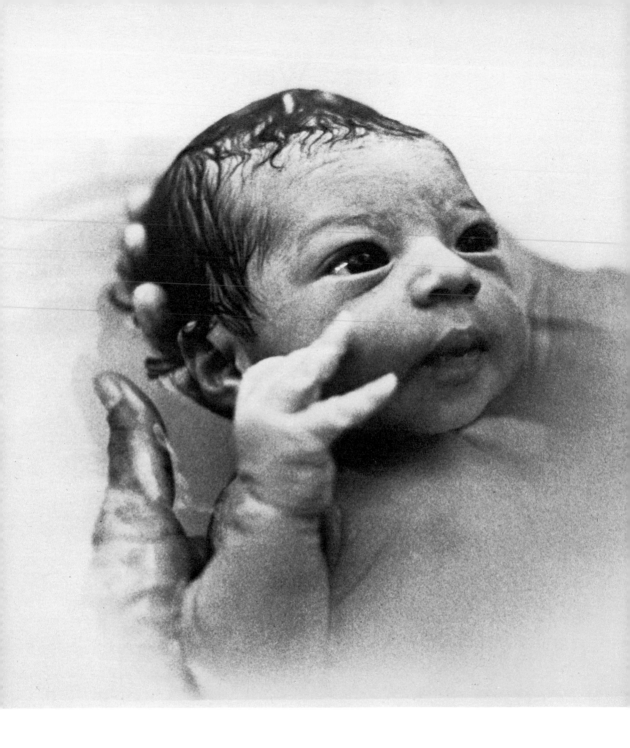

A new world! and the undrugged baby is awake and aware to meet it and to get to know its parents from the very first moments. •With the help of a doctor or midwife the mother can put her hands down and lift her baby out of her own body. The child opens its eyes and meets its mother's. They are face to face. •A partnership has already started.

Forty Weeks

Reflections & Observations

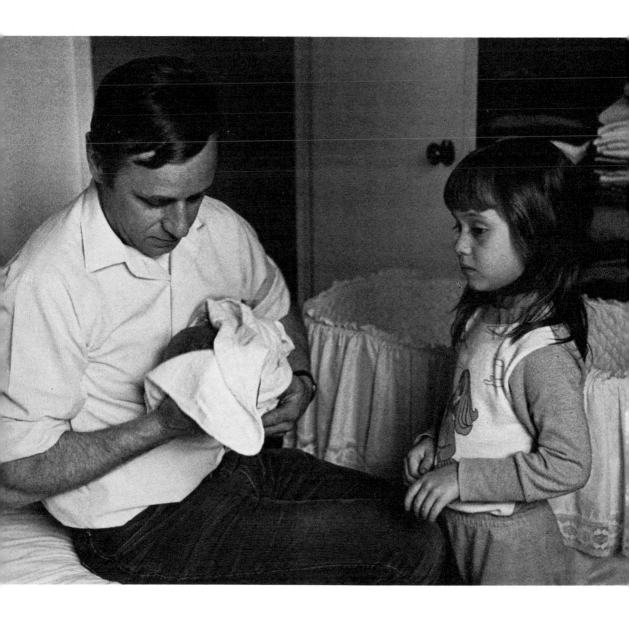

First Week after Birth

When a baby is pushed out into the world it is not only that a child is born, but in that moment also a mother and father start to be born. •The birth of a child is the birth of a family. For this to happen you need to be in an environment which offers you close contact and time to get to know each other. Cuddle your baby, talk to her, let her know she is welcome and that there are arms to hold and make a safe haven for her. Take the baby into bed with you so that she is aware of your steady heartbeat and the comforting sounds she was already used to in your uterus. Keep her warm with the warmth flowing from your own body. Create opportunities for other members of the family to enjoy the baby, too. •And if there are already other children changes are bound to take place in the relationship between each member of the family. The process of change can be a difficult transition for each one, especially for older brothers and sisters who can no longer be babies, perhaps sometimes before they are quite ready to grow up. This challenge offers an opportunity to grow emotionally. The birth of a baby can be a developmental experience.

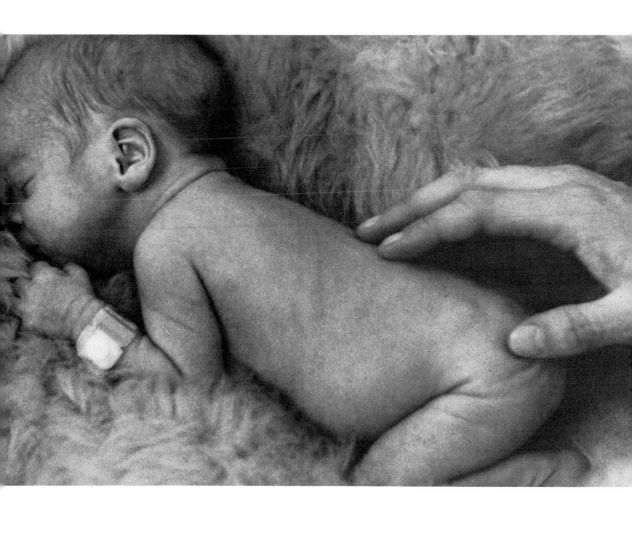

Second Week after Birth

Your body is undergoing dramatic changes. It is empty of the baby and you may feel lost without a baby inside you. How different is the baby from the one you imagined? It is sometimes difficult to relate the reality of the baby in your arms to the baby who was in the uterus. It often takes time to get to know and like the surprising little creature who has put in an appearance if you had imagined you were having a very different baby, even, perhaps, one of the other sex. The child inside you was automatically nourished and cared for. But now you have to come to terms with a new person who seeks your undivided attention and whose very presence forces you to acquire new skills. There is for many women a spontaneous grieving after birth because of this separation. •Put the baby in a carrier snuggled against your body and the closeness will help you feel whole again, as well as being comforting and familiar for the baby, who has to cope with the same separation from your body. •It can be painful to rediscover your changed body, not pregnant and full any more, yet not as it was before you conceived, soft, damp, leaking lochia and milk, like a moist, ripe fruit, a body which has opened wide and released the baby and is not yet closed up again, firm in its boundaries. You may feel very vulnerable, tender, exposed and rather bruised, and this not just physically but psychologically. •Take some time to get to know your new body. Your breasts may be aching, but it feels good to have your back stroked. You are probably very aware of your crumpled, flabby abdomen and don't find this an attractive part of your body to focus on, but neck, shoulder and foot massage help you relax. •The best exercises are rhythmic ones in which you are not forced to hold your breath because of the effort you are putting into them. Movements should be flowing and full, not jerky and strained. Lying on a firm surface with one pillow under your head and your knees bent and drawn up near your buttocks, take a complete breath in, allowing your abdomen to swell up, and then give a long, long breath out, sucking in your abdominal wall, pulling it towards your spine. •Then blow out through pursed lips any remaining breath as if you were blowing out a candle and draw in your abdominal wall still further as you do so. When you are ready to take another breath let the abdomen swell up again and go on breathing rhythmically like this for twenty breaths. Plan several sessions of this breathing at set times of the day and your abdominal muscles will recover their tone. •Even more important than exercises is your posture right through each day. Tighten your buttocks when you stand up, walk tall, check the way you are standing sideways-on in a full-length mirror. Carry the baby in a sling rather than on your hip so that you don't twist your spine. •Feed the baby with your feet up whenever possible and if it is small put a pillow on your lap and rest it on it so that you do not slump forward with shoulders and breasts dragged down. See that your back is well supported with an extra cushion if necessary. Relax your shoulders, with elbows dropped out rather than clamped to your sides and use an extra cushion if you need it for your arm to rest on. Practice your relaxation, which is as important for you and your baby now as it was in labour. •When picking up anything from the floor, making a bed or cleaning the bath, use your knees and bend your legs, not your back. Walk vigorously, with long strides, arms swinging, the best exercise of all. Sit rather than stand and whenever you have a choice between sitting and lying, lie down.

First and Second Weeks
after Birth

Reflections & Observations

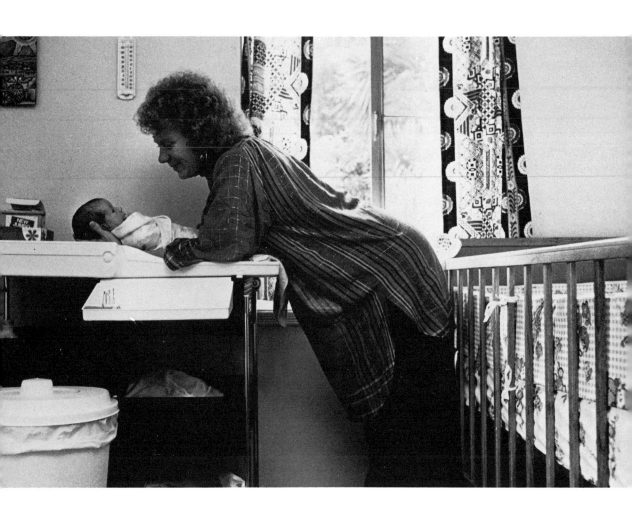

Third Week after Birth

A feeling of let-down after the 'high' of the birth is natural. Though you may have expected it to come three or four days after the birth it often does not occur till later and is common any time within the first month. •Let yourself weep. You'll get over it quicker that way. The worst thing you can do is to try and bottle up the emotions and struggle bravely on. •You are probably short of sleep. Fatigue makes you more emotional. Lie down and relax whenever you can, even if it is not yet lunchtime. You will feel all the better for it. Many new babies sleep solidly in the morning after being restless through the night. They have not yet developed their diurnal rhythms. Take the opportunity of getting some rest yourself. •Being a mother, especially for the first time, is hard work. Everything that you will later do automatically, without having to think about it, you now do laboriously, slowly, painstakingly, and even then you're not sure you've done it right. •The skills of changing nappies without fussing the baby too much, of putting a vest on deftly, of bathing the baby so that it doesn't scream all the time (after feeding is the answer, not before) do not come naturally just because you are now a mother. They have to be learned and at first you probably feel all thumbs. Your partner feels like this too. So learn together. Each parent can acquire the new skills and get to know their baby better as they do so. •It doesn't matter that you are inefficient at first. The important thing is to give the baby good experiences and the sense of security and trust that comes with this. The baby will quickly let you know what these good experiences are, so learn from your baby and you are on the way to developing a warm, loving relationship even though you haven't got the techniques right.

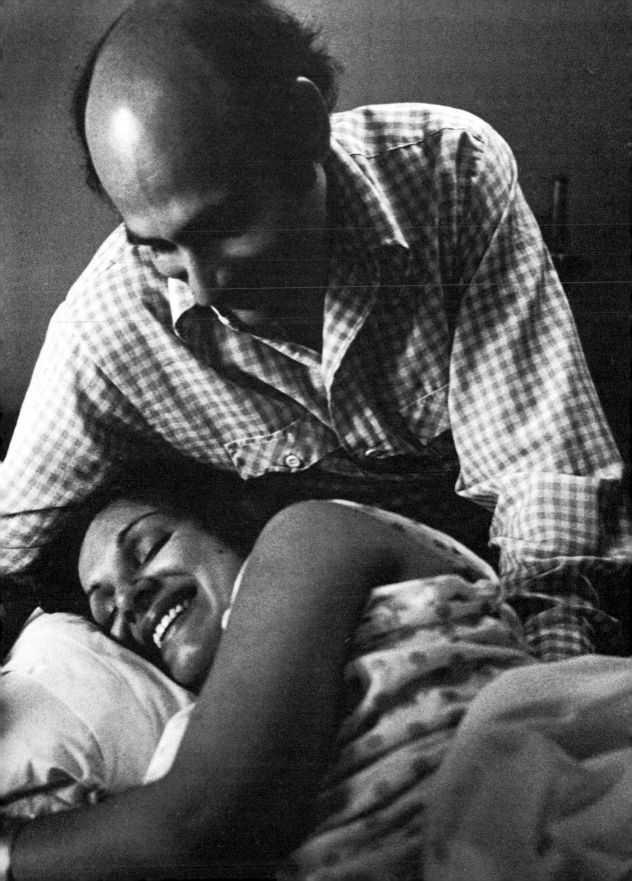

Fourth Week after Birth

Make love whenever you feel you want to. There is no need to wait until after the postnatal examination. If you have had an episiotomy, or if the tissues have torn, entry may still be painful at this time but once your partner's penis is deep inside it should not hurt, provided that he does not put any weight on the area of scar tissue, which is usually the part of the vagina nearest the anus. You will find that pillows are useful to avoid directing friction or pressure against this area. ●You may notice at first that you are slow to lubricate. Normally with sexual excitement all the walls of the vagina become moistened, and it is important that your partner does not enter if you are dry. He can gently spread a lubricating cream or lotion with a finger before the actual penetration. After stimulating you with his fingers it is most comfortable if he just slips inside and then waits so that you draw his penis further in with your own pelvic-floor muscles. These muscles may be slack at first but will get stronger and more active the more you use them. ●To be pleasurable sex should not be goal-orientated. There is no goal to be achieved, and lovemaking can be enjoyable with or without orgasm.
●You may discover that milk shoots from your nipples during lovemaking. Some couples don't like it and if you feel this way, have a towel handy. Others enjoy it as an exciting part of lovemaking. If you do not feel ready for full lovemaking, enjoy pleasuring each other and let genital feelings be gradually aroused.
●It is often forgotten that the coming of a baby can be just as intense and moving an experience for the father as it is for the mother. The man may be caught in the currents of deep and far-reaching emotions at the time of birth and afterwards. These emotions, the 'highs' and the 'lows', give special meaning to the relationship with the woman who is the mother of his child and affect the way he feels about the newborn. Invisible bonds tie him to his baby just as securely as they unite mother and baby.

Third and Fourth Weeks
after Birth

Reflections & Observations

Fifth Week after Birth

Cuddle your baby whenever you want to. You can't 'spoil' newborn babies. They thrive emotionally by being kissed and cuddled just as they thrive physically on their mother's milk. ●The relationship between a mother and her baby need not be an exclusive one. It is enriched by sharing and when all three, mother, father and baby, enjoy each other together. You are concentrating now on looking after your baby. But it is vital that you also look after yourself. Even with babies who feed regularly every three or four hours, by the time you have put them down the space between feedings is only two or three hours. And many have very irregular hunger pangs in the first six weeks, (they settle into a rhythm after that). ●Use the time when you know that the baby is most likely to be asleep to get sleep yourself, *not* to do the laundry. ●Don't be afraid to take your baby into bed with you. You won't roll over on it unless you are heavily sedated or drunk, and the skin contact between you is good for both. ●Make sure you are eating enough and getting sufficient protein foods, fruit and vegetables. You need 500–1000 extra calories when breastfeeding in the form of dairy products and other types of protein, whole grains, salads and fresh fruit. ●Keep a pile of books by your bed for those really long drawn-out feedings or listen to music. Make your bed or a couch a centre of luxury and relaxation which you, your baby, and your partner can enjoy together. ●Your postnatal examination probably takes place next week. Make a list of anything you want to discuss with the doctor before you go.

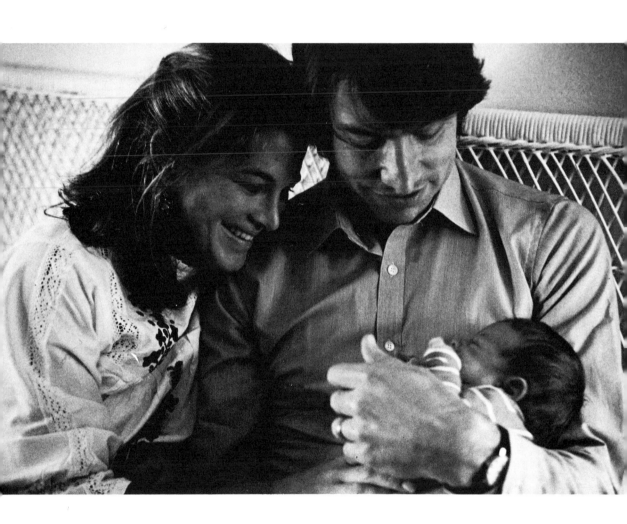

Sixth Week after Birth

You're quite right if you think that your baby has been able to see ever since you first met. Babies can see at birth and can even follow a moving shape, though they can focus only on a spot about eight inches away from their faces. When you hold your baby in your arms for a feed this is just the distance from your face. Many newborn babies fall asleep as soon as their tummies are full, but as they get older they are often alert and watchful for minutes at a time after eating and it is then that you notice your baby staring at your face. •Research shows that babies like complicated shapes to look at with pattern and texture and different dimensions. Best of all they like the human face and your baby has already learned a lot about you by studying you carefully and certainly knows you. At about this time the baby moves its head and eyes to follow shapes up and down and sideways. You can test this when the baby is in a quiet, alert state by holding an interesting object like a bright Christmas tree ornament or a rattle where the baby can focus on it, and then slowly moving it up and down from side to side. •Your baby can interact with the environment and learn through seeing much better when propped up than when lying flat in a carry-cot or pram. •Around this time, too, the baby begins to look pleased and to smile when enjoying things, usually in response to your face and voice, and starts to make the cooing sound which is the beginning of speech. •To get to know your baby better watch carefully to see what things produce the concentrated attention which then blossoms into a smile.

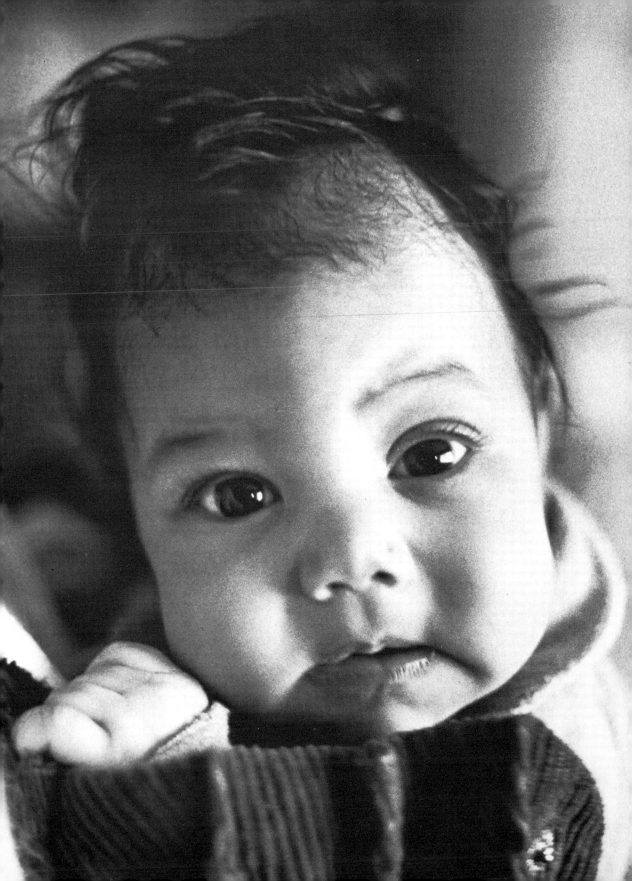

Fifth and Sixth Weeks
after Birth

Reflections & Observations

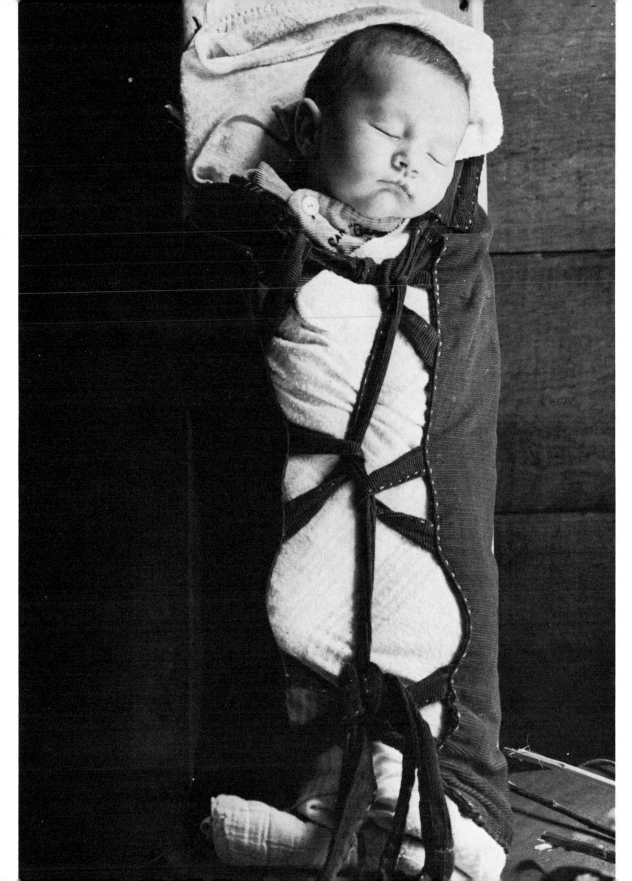

Seventh Week after Birth

In many cultures babies are bound with strips of cloth or animal skin to a cradle, board, or the mother's body. Babies seem to sleep best when firmly held, or even swaddled, in the early weeks. Perhaps this re-creates the sense of being hugged by the walls of the uterus. •They also like being rocked, which resembles the regular rocking movement of your pelvis as you walked during pregnancy. And they are soothed by the rumble of a washing machine or dishwasher or the hum of a vacuum cleaner, a car or the radio. In fact a baby may sleep much more soundly with a background of steady noise or human conversation than in silence. •They like being patted on the bottom too, with a steady beat like the beat of your heart, another familiar feeling. If your baby finds it hard to drift into sleep, try patting like this. •Some like sleeping on their sides; some prefer to be on their fronts, head turned to the side. This is a good position if your baby tends to bring back milk, as the milk can't then get down into the windpipe. •Find out what helps your baby to settle most easily, but remember that babies do get as much sleep as they need, even if *you* could do with more. They haven't read the books about how much sleep experts think they ought to have. And, whatever the theories, you cannot *make* a baby sleep. •It is useful to discover your baby's sleep pattern as it helps you to find some pattern in your own day. You can use the squares on this page. Shade in the half-hour periods when the baby is sleeping over three days and even if it seemed chaotic you will find that a pattern is emerging.

DAY ONE

DAY TWO

DAY THREE

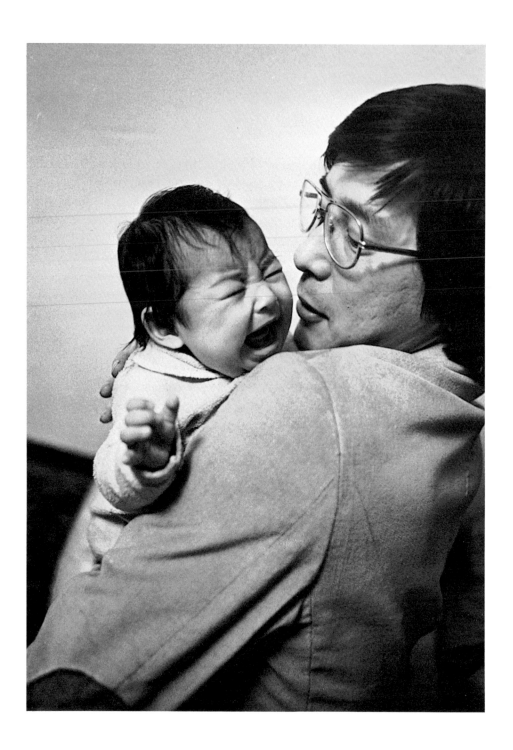

Eighth Week after Birth

Babies send messages with different kinds of crying. You will have learned by now that your baby's crying varies according to whether he or she is hungry, thirsty, tired, bored, lonely, cold or in pain. As you understand your baby's language better you will be able to interpret these different cries with more certainty. Let your feelings guide you. •It doesn't do any good for a baby to go on crying and it certainly doesn't 'exercise the lungs.' A baby who is allowed to cry for a long time may become too overwrought or exhausted to be able to feed, and then cries from hunger and thirst. •Babies cry because they need to be held and cuddled and to hear your voice and have human contact. They are not being naughty when they do this. They are crying for love and attention, not just for food. Nestling your baby in a sling close to your body is comforting for both of you. Some mothers find that their babies are soothed by massage. Some soothe their babies by singing to them. People often say that babies have 'colic' when in fact they are needing comfort and human contact or are simply bored. Around twelve weeks this kind of crying tends to stop and babies seem to be able to amuse themselves better. •At about this time you may notice that your baby will lie awake sometimes quite happily provided that there is something interesting to look at. •If you ignore or are slow to respond to your baby's crying research shows that the baby is more likely to become a persistent crier and to be difficult to handle at one year old. Mothers who are quick to pick up their babies keep them close, and feed them when they cry are most likely to have one-year-olds who are easy. The baby of a responsive mother learns trust. •There come times when you may feel angry or desperate and you can't stand the baby's crying or fussing any longer and that you must get away. Whereas most of the time you respond to the baby's crying with tenderness and concern, if you are under stress the responsibility for this new, completely dependent creature can be very threatening, or the baby may seem so rejecting and hostile to you personally that you feel attacked by the cries. There is nothing abnormal about feeling sometimes that you have had enough. Perhaps your partner or a neighbour or friend can take the baby while you have a break. All mothers need space between them and their children occasionally, just to belong to themselves for a while.

Seventh and Eighth Weeks
after Birth

Reflections & Observations

Ninth Week after Birth

Conversations with your baby start long before speech. As with any conversation it involves turn-taking. You smile and see that the baby is starting to get interested and then the baby bursts into a lovely smile. The baby copies the movements of your mouth as you talk too. If you purse your lips or stick out your tongue the baby will probably copy you, even if in a rather rudimentary way. The baby uses his hands to accompany the speech patterns too, just as adults do. •If you talk to a baby too vigorously and too long and never give the baby a turn he may get fretful and cry. It's important to be quiet and look away occasionally and let the baby have a chance to have a share in the conversation. •Talking to your baby is important because she learns how to become an active partner in a relationship and this leads later on to all the skills of living in society. •At about this age the baby finds her hands. At first it happens by chance as the waving hands pass her field of vision. But then she discovers that she can do exciting things with them. If you fix a rattle or beads to the cot he learns that he can bang them and produce a pleasing noise. The extension of the ability to 'hold' with the eyes to being able to grasp and retain with the hands is a marvellous discovery for the baby. When you breastfeed you may find that the baby grabs on to your breast or to a strand of your hair or your clothing with a tight little hand.

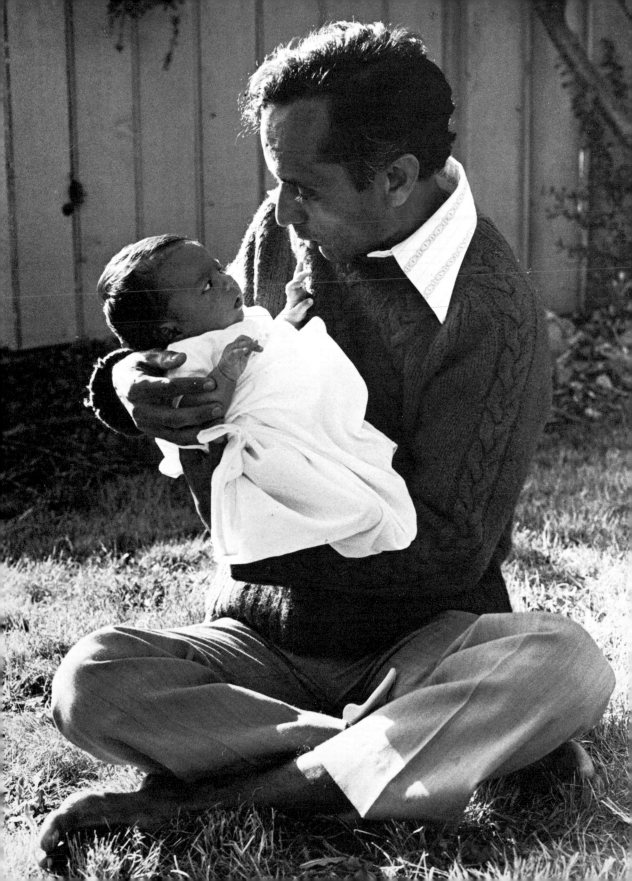

Tenth Week after Birth

Postnatal exercises are important to restore muscle tone. As your baby grows you will find you are constantly carrying a heavy weight, and your muscles need to be in good shape. Lying on your back, arms stretched above your head, flatten your wrist against the floor, and pull in your tummy muscles, without holding your breath. Now swing your right leg up and over your body, and stretch it out straight as far as it will on the other side. Then lift it and swing it back in the same way. Now do the same with your left leg. Continue doing the movement rhythmically, starting five times each side and working up to ten times each side. This exercise is good for the waist, thighs and tummy muscles. •Another good way of firming tummy muscles is belly dancing, either with or without music. Keep your shoulders still and move your pelvis in circles and you'll feel your tummy and buttock muscles and leg muscles contracting and releasing. •If you can attend postnatal exercise classes you also meet other new mothers, and sharing the experience of new parenthood can be rewarding. In some areas postnatal support groups arrange swimming sessions in pools which are specially heated so that you can take your baby and toddler in with you. •Swimming, vigorous walking and dancing are all excellent kinds of movement to get your figure back. And it is particularly important to exercise the muscles of the pelvic floor which support your uterus and bladder. These are the muscles around your vagina and anus and further up inside and it is important to tone them by tightening them at regular intervals. •Contract these muscles several times whenever you change a nappy, do dishes, ride in a lift, wait in the super-market checkout line or for the traffic lights to change when you are in a car. Gradually you will find that you can hold these muscles tight for longer and longer without discomfort and without the muscles starting to tremble.

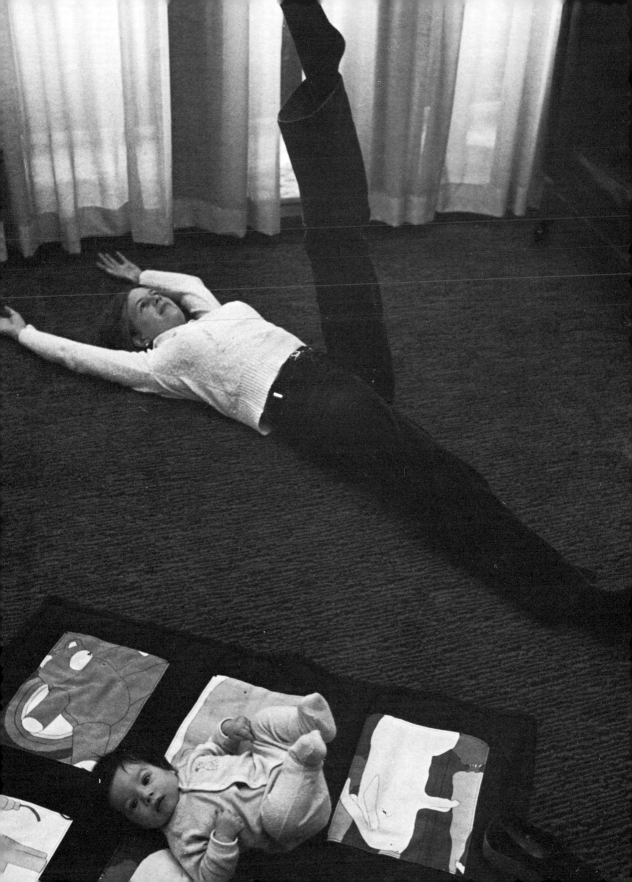

Ninth and Tenth Weeks
after Birth

Reflections & Observations

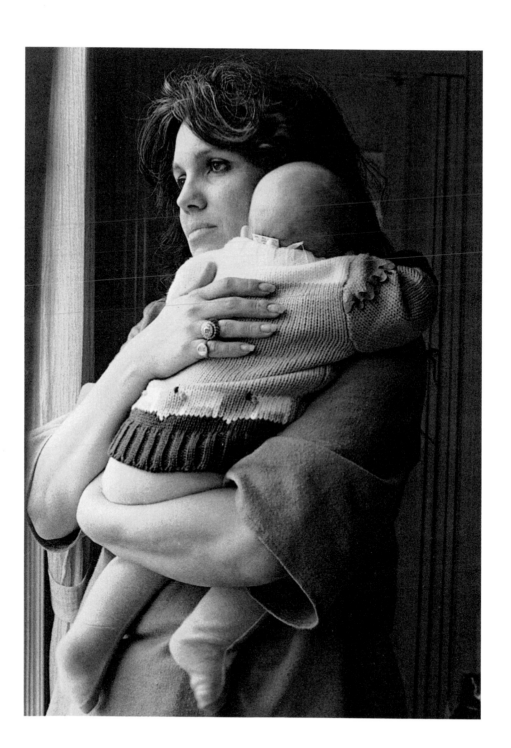

Eleventh Week after Birth

There often comes a time when a woman begins to wonder if she is beginning to lose touch with the world. Is she capable only of baby talk? Sometimes this grows into a feeling of deep resentment against the baby who has 'trapped' you into motherhood. •Talk with your partner about this. Is it possible to have a baby sitter sometimes? Could you get together with other couples who have babies? Can you arrange a babysitting co-op so that couples can get out together in the evenings? •Meals out, car rides, long country walks, picnics can all be done with the baby. It may not be easy to organize these things but you are husband and wife and lovers as well as parents. •It is good for both you and your baby if another loving person is able to take over the baby's care for short periods, even if it is only long enough for you to have a nap or a luxuriously long bath. If this is difficult to manage, you can at least arrange to meet another mother and baby regularly so that you have some adult conversation and your baby gets a chance to meet another person about the same size. •At about this time babies uncurl from their fetal position and are happy to lie on their tummies on a rug spread on the floor in a warm room and exercise their limbs. They push their feet against your hands, bob their heads up and look about, and even lift their shoulders right up. If you put a baby down on his side he will be able to roll over on his back. If you put him on his back, he will wave arms and legs about. The opportunity to explore different positions and types of body movement is important for the baby. It is very dull for any baby to be left for long periods lying flat on her back or wrapped up tightly like a sausage. No wonder babies who are treated like this get very bored!

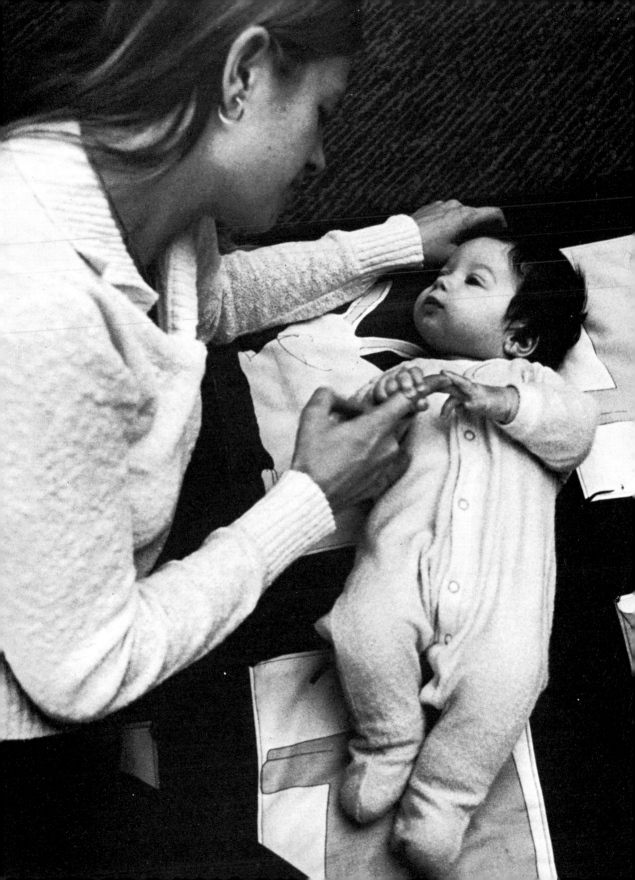

Twelfth Week after Birth

At about this time many babies seem to get tired of doing nothing and are restless unless they are stimulated and given some entertainment. You may think it is hunger at first and wonder whether you have enough milk, but then discover that your baby isn't solely interested in feeding and begins to play during a feed. •Use your imagination to provide the baby with a variety of different things to see, hear and touch. If you have an inclined baby seat or bouncer with good back support the baby gets a different view of the world. The seat can be propped on a kitchen counter or draining board, but see that it is stable and well away from hot water taps, kettles, saucepans and electric outlets and plugs. As your baby becomes more mobile and waves its arms and legs about you need to think ahead about possible dangers, like hot cups of coffee within range, too. •Rig up a variety of differently shaped, sized and coloured objects on a string or rubber band in front of the baby where they can be kicked or handled. Change them every now and again. •When you can sit down place the baby on your lap and read the newspaper or a magazine or book. Babies are interested in the patterns of newsprint and especially the pictures. •Take time off to play with your baby and enjoy each other. A father gets a lot out of playing with his baby too, even at this age. There is no reason why a woman should *instinctively* be able to know what to do for a small baby with any more accuracy than a man. A father who is used to doing things for the baby and who has got to really know her as a person, gives a great deal to his child, and also gains much. In spite of the common assumption that men are too rough and tough to care for a newborn, you only have to think how tender your man can be in lovemaking to realize that the same tenderness can be expressed towards his baby.

Eleventh and Twelfth Weeks
after Birth

Reflections & Observations

Afterword

And so it will go on, from day to day and week to week, fascinating things to learn about your baby, a new adventure for both of you. The basis of this is watching and learning from the baby and never getting stuck with unthinking responses to behaviour which is constantly changing as he or she develops. Your interaction with your baby is unique, like an intricate dance to an entirely new melody which you are working out together. At times you will miss a step or two and then again find a satisfying rhythm. •When you feel you are making a bad job of it, remember that becoming a mother takes time, that it is a *process* rather than an act. You will find, too, that the way you mother changes as your baby develops. A woman who is a good mother for a newborn baby isn't a good one for a five- or six-month-old unless she changes and grows along with her baby. The same goes for fathers, too. Being parents is a great education! •Far in the future, when your child asks you to tell about the beginning of her or his life, you will have this record of your thoughts and feelings at the time. Children are fascinated by the story of the start of their own lives, the shadowy beginnings before the curtain went up on self-consciousness and verbal memory. Now you have created the basis on which you can describe this period vividly and honestly.

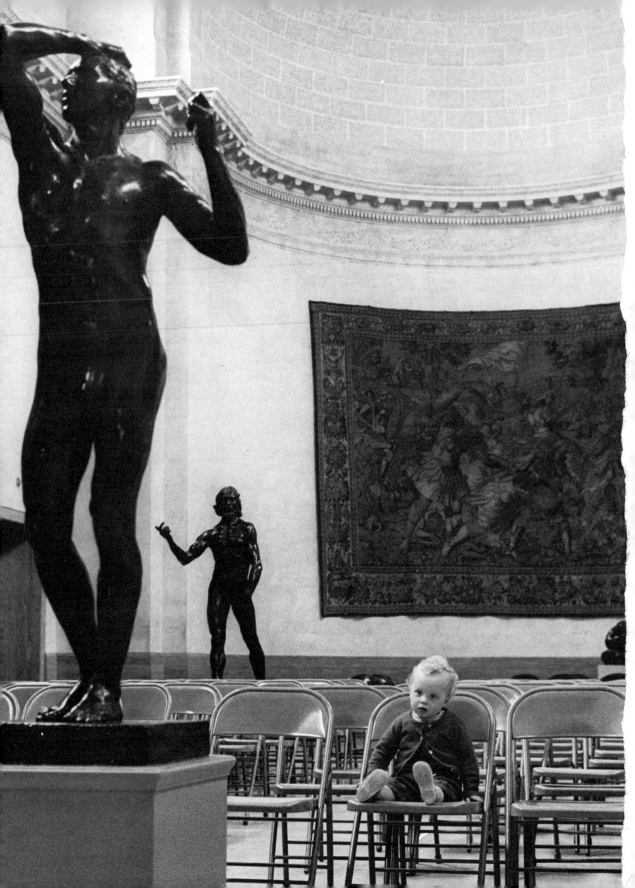